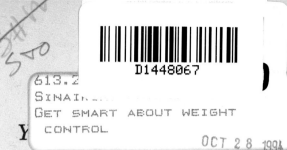
Y

"Dieting is the *only* way to lose weight!"

"Identifying food allergies
can help you get in shape."

"If you want to stay slim,
there are some foods
you just can't have."

"You can spot reduce with special exercises."

Now learn the *facts* . . .

GET SMART ABOUT
WEIGHT CONTROL

Also by Phillip M. Sinaikin, M.D.
(with Judith Sachs)

FAT MADNESS
AFTER THE FAST

Most Berkley Books are available at special quantity discounts for bulk purchases for sales promotions, premiums, fundraising, or educational use. Special books or book excerpts can also be created to fit specific needs.

For details, write or telephone Special Markets, The Berkley Publishing Group, 200 Madison Avenue, New York, New York 10016; (212) 951-8891.

GET SMART ABOUT WEIGHT CONTROL

HOW TO DEVELOP YOUR OWN
LIFELONG WEIGHT CONTROL PROGRAM

PHILLIP M. SINAIKIN, M.D.

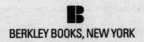

BERKLEY BOOKS, NEW YORK

GET SMART ABOUT WEIGHT CONTROL

A Berkley Book / published by arrangement with
PIA Specialty Press, Inc.

PRINTING HISTORY
PIA Press edition published 1988
Berkley edition / August 1994

ISBN: 0-425-13763-5

BERKLEY®
Berkley Books are published by The Berkley Publishing Group,
200 Madison Avenue, New York, New York 10016.
BERKLEY and the "B" design
are trademarks belonging to Berkley Publishing Corporation.

PRINTED IN THE UNITED STATES OF AMERICA

10 9 8 7 6 5 4 3 2 1

The author gratefully acknowledges the assistance of Anne Edelstein in the writing and preparation of this book.

Grateful acknowledgment is made to the following for the right to reprint or adapt previously published material:

"Summary of Popular Dietary Approaches to Weight Control," Cherly L. Rock, M.M.Sc., R.D., and Ann M. Coulston, *Journal of The American Dietetic Association*, v. 88, no. 1, Jan. 1988.

"Comparison of Diets to Dieting Goals," Dr. Paul La Chance, Michelle C. Fischer, R.D., Rutgers University, 1983.

"Exercise Program Compliance," Barry A. Franklin, Ph.D., *Behavioral Management of Obesity,* edited by JS Storlie and HA Jordan, Spectrum Publications, Inc., Jamaica, NY, 1984.

"Calories Used Per Minute During Activity," Human Performances Research Center, Brigham Young University.

"1980 Metropolitan Height & Weight Tables," Metropolitan Life Insurance Co.

New American Eating Guide, Center for Science in the Public Interest, 1501 16th St. N.W., Washington, DC. 20036.

Contents

To my inspiration, guide, and love of my life,
Ronnie, and our three daughters:
Jamie, Benay, and Shara.

Preface

"The three letter words are worse than the
four letter words. And the worst of all is
F-A-T."

Those immortal words were uttered by 66-year-
old actress Olivia de Havilland after a three week,
$4,725 stay at a plush fat farm outside of San
Francisco. Her money bought an 800 calorie a day
diet, exercise routines from morning to night, special lotions and body wraps, and a net 12 pound
weight loss. While few of us can afford $393 per
pound to lose weight, if we had it, most of us would
pay it!

As a physician and a psychiatrist, I'm often
amazed at the lengths people are willing to go to
lose weight, even if they have other, more serious
issues to deal with. Most of the time, these patients of mine truly believe that they only can be
happy if they are as thin as the models they see
in magazines and on TV. If they can get as thin
as they think they should be, they'll gain admi-
ration, self-esteem, occupational potential, re-
spect, love.......HAPPINESS!

My patients, like millions more, are victims of a sort of "fat madness" that leads them to these mistaken beliefs. The constant reinforcement by the media of this belief makes it very hard to convince them that "thinness" won't buy happiness.

But, there is an answer for people who are caught on a diet merry-go-round and can't get off. I've written this book to give everyone the only weapon they really need to both lose weight, and retain their sanity.

That weapon is the truth.

This book gives the reader accurate information about diet, exercise, nutrition, and weight control that will enable him or her to create a weight-loss program that fits their own lifestyle—not that of a "diet guru." By understanding why current myths are just that—false beliefs, the reader can make diet and exercise choices based on medical realities, not media hyped "magic" packages.

Getting thin should not be an all-consuming goal. What you have to do is put your weight loss desires into a rational context. And you can begin that process by getting smart—learning the truth and the facts as explained in this book.

It's my belief that everyone can lose weight if they need to and still be happy, even if they don't end up looking like a fashion model. Once you've read the information in this book, you'll be an educated consumer, and you'll be on your way.

—Phillip M. Sinaikin, M.D.

The Truth About Weight Control

While we still don't understand everything about weight control, science has proved one important fact: there is no magic way to control our weight. The miracle cure—the painless method to lose weight that we've been waiting for—simply *does not exist*. The principles that *will* keep us healthy and fit involve nutrition, exercise, and body chemistry. There simply is no easy solution. But this is not necessarily bad news: Science has also taught us how to control weight without jeopardizing our health. That's what you can learn to do when you read this book.

First a note of caution. Getting smart about weight control takes a little effort. But once you get "into the process" and become involved in learning the facts about diet and weight loss, it won't be long before you have a weight control program that works. The best part about this process—which is really an educational one—is that it doesn't require buying expensive fad diet foods, numerous diet books or even radically changing your life-style.

If it's so easy, you might ask, why can't everybody weigh what they want, and stop following the newest diet guru to appear on the TV talk show circuit?

One reason is that people resist the truth, especially when glamorous or exciting personalities say that anyone can be like they are. Another is that educating people about new developments in medical science has never been an easy task. The scientists, researchers, and physicians trying to inform the public about the truth about weight control face a difficult task. What we are up against are misguided myths, which have been promoted to support a very lucrative diet industry that harms many more people than it helps.

The hard truth is that dieting alone will not control weight. More than 90 percent of all dieters gain back the weight they've lost within two years. And despite the hundreds of diet programs developed every year, no single approach has worked consistently over time for the majority of people. The reality is that we live in a world of weight control myths and fantasies—a world created by our emotional investment in being thin and our willingness to spend endless sums of money trying to lose weight.

Unfortunately, we *will* continue to be victimized by fad weight loss schemes; we *will* continue to be seduced by one outlandish diet after another, continually falling prey to programs that get us to lose weight only to gain it right back again. We will continue, that is, unless we are able to do one simple thing: *Get Smart About Weight Control!*

We *can* stop torturing ourselves. We *can* lead lives that are free from failed diets and guilt-ridden binges. But in order to do this, we must learn and accept the scientific facts about weight control. And that is exactly what this book will help you do!

In the following pages we will examine commonly held myths and fantasies about weight control, health, current fads, and social issues. We will explode these myths, uncovering the reasons for their existence and continued popularity. And then we will replace them with the truth.

OUR REAL "NATIONAL PASTIME"

Weight control has become a national obsession. In a society in which we painstakingly save every penny just to pay the mortgage and make ends meet—in which we elect leaders based on their promises to keep our taxes down—we nonetheless willingly spend more than 15 *billion* dollars a year on weight control. Eagerly we throw our money away on diet books, diet clinics, diet foods, exercise plans, pills, and lotions, all promising the same thing: that we will be thin.

One of the side effects of our thinness obsession

WHERE DO YOU FIT IN?

In February 1984 *Glamour* magazine published the results of a fascinating survey of 33,000 women and their attitudes about themselves and their attitudes toward their weight. Take a moment and ask yourself how you would fit in this survey (the results of the *Glamour* survey are in the figures in the parentheses.)

Which would make you happiest?
- **A)** A date with a man you admire?   (21%)
- **B)** Success at work?   (22%)
- **C)** Losing weight?   (42%)
- **D)** Hearing from an old friend?   (15%)

Does weight affect how you think about yourself?
- **A)** Often   (63%)
- **B)** Sometimes   (33%)
- **C)** Never   (4%)

How happy are you with your body?
- **A)** Very happy   (6%)
- **B)** Moderately happy   (53%)
- **C)** Moderately unhappy   (30%)
- **D)** Very unhappy   (11%)

Do you feel:
- **A)** just right?   (15%)
- **B)** too thin?   (3%)
- **C)** too fat?   (75%)
- **D)** too short?   (6%)
- **E)** too tall?   (1%)

What often triggers overeating?
- **A)** loneliness/boredom   (62%)

B) depression (44%)
C) stress/anxiety (34%)

Are you self conscious about your body?
   A) Around almost anyone (46%)
   B) Mainly around men (27%)
   C) Almost never (19%)
   D) Mainly around women (5%)
   E) Mainly around family (3%)

How do you feel about these parts of your body:

	PROUD/ SATISFIED	DISSATISFIED/ ASHAMED
Breasts	71%	29%
Stomach	36%	64%
Hips	39%	61%
Thighs	28%	72%
Calves	77%	23%
Feet	81%	19%

Which of the following have you used to control your weight?

	NEVER	SOMETIMES	OFTEN
Moderate calorie restric- tion	12%	41%	47%
Crash diets	42%	40%	18%
Liquid- formula diet	73%	22%	5%
Exercise	5%	38%	57%
Diet pills	50%	38%	12%
Laxatives	82%	14%	4%
Diuretics	82%	14%	4%
Fasting/ starving	55%	34%	11%
Self- induced vomiting	85%	10%	5%

is an alarming increase in eating disorders like bulimia and anorexia. Young children are stunting their growth by going on rigorous diets before their bones have fully developed. Teenagers and adults measure their self-esteem on a daily basis by a number on a scale, determining their self-worth by their capacity to endure starvation.

Where did this obsession come from? Why has thinness become the stepping-stone to beauty, happiness, and "the good life". The weight loss "game" is actually not a new phenomenon. Society has always been obsessed with physical appearance. At different times in our history, fat was "in," and women strived for the voluptuous, Rubenesque-type of body, considered to be a paragon of beauty. Yet in Victorian times, some women actually had their lower ribs *removed,* so that they could tighten their corsets as much as possible without piercing their livers!

Today, our preoccupation with thinness has been encouraged by the media. Turn on the TV, flip through a magazine, go to the movies—the virtues and desirability of being thin are constantly paraded before us. Role models and heroes of the past, such as the voluptuous Mae West, have been replaced by rail-thin superstars like Christie Brinkley and Michael Jackson. The message is quite clear: Be thin and you, too, can be popular, sexually fulfilled, and successful. After all, how many overweight athletes, movie stars, and other glamorous role models are there? It's no wonder that, despite the odds against it, we all want to be thin.

THE AGE OF THE DIET GURU

Let's talk about "diet gurus." These "experts" tell us that for a price we can: lose weight while sleeping; lose ten pounds in seven days; lose weight while eating all we want. "New speak" terms, such as *food combinations, food allergies,* and *food addictions,* have quickly become part of our vocabulary. The "gurus" who use these terms have convinced us because we want to believe in a simple answer, as consumers, we have accepted the myth, the big lie, that it is easy to lose weight quickly, safely, and permanently. Undaunted by repeated failures, we keep coming back for more, buying one new product or diet after another. How can a physician—advising on proper nutrition, exercise, genetics, and metabolism—possibly compete with this diet mania?

It's not easy, but I'm determined to try, if you are!

The first thing I tell my patients about is the importance of understanding the truth about weight control. A thorough understanding of these facts is the single most important step you can take in formulating a safe, sane, and effective means of controlling your weight. This informed approach has been made more effective by recent scientific research. Scientists still don't fully understand the very complex subject of body weight regulation. But new research is providing us with valuable tools to aid in constructing a weight control program.

GET STARTED TODAY

Knowledge is power. If you learn the real facts about weight control, you can free yourself from the diet traps that have poisoned your perceptions about your body weight. Then, after reading this book, you'll be able to employ your new knowledge to design your own long-term weight control program, a program suited to your individual needs and realities. This time your diet and your behavior will not be undermined by false beliefs and promises, but instead will be guided by sound scientific principles that will help you get your weight where it should be and keep it there.

What's different about this book? Well, for one thing, the first step I recommend is to do *nothing,* except to learn some real facts about losing and understanding weight. So, enroll yourself in Get Smart About Weight Control's first class. By the end of the chapter 5 you'll be amazed and maybe even shocked at how different the reality is from the myths we've come to believe about dieting.

The Myths About Dieting and Exercising

MYTH: DIETING IS THE BEST WAY TO LOSE WEIGHT

In fact, dieting may be the *worst* way to lose weight and the *best* way to gain weight!

That's ridiculous, you're saying. Common sense tells us that if overeating causes fatness, then undereating should make us thinner. But common sense can be misleading—after all, anyone with a weight problem knows through personal experience that "dieting" leads to weight loss. However, the constant dieter also knows deep down that, in the long run, "going on a diet" doesn't always work. The vast majority of people who lose weight by dieting alone gain it back again. Understanding why "dieting" fails is the most important step we can take on the road to an intelligent weight control program.

WHOSE FAULT IS IT?

Most people believe that the reason their diet fails is their own failure to stick to it exactly—going off on an eating binge, for example. Are they weak? Is this true? The answer is a reassuring *No*.

Dieting is a complex physiological process that can best be understood by the following equation:

**Energy Consumed − Energy Expended =
Body Fat (Gained or Lost)**

Simply put, this means that if the Energy Consumed (i.e., the food we eat) exceeds the Energy Expended or burned up, then we will gain body fat. Body fat is lost when Energy Consumed is less than the Energy Expended. According to this, then dieting should work. But unfortunately, life is not that simple. What science has uncovered complicates this seemingly simple equation. We know that energy expenditure is the "monkey wrench" that disrupts the equation, and causes diets to fail.

Energy expenditure consists of three components. The first, and the most important, component is *basal metabolism*—the energy required to run the body when it's at rest. The energy needed to keep our hearts beating, our lungs working, and countless other essential bodily functions operating makes up our basal metabolism. Basal metabolism accounts for 50 to 70 percent of our daily energy expenditure.

The second component of energy expenditure is physical activity (couch potatoes, beware!). The amount of calories expended is directly related to the intensity and duration of the exercise. Everything counts: walking up steps, hammering a nail, washing clothes, even sex. (Did you know that overweight people often have a higher calorie requirement for physical activity; heavier people have more weight to move around, and they burn off more calories in the process.) Physical activity accounts for 25 to 40 percent of our daily energy expenditure.

The third and final component is the energy required to digest the food we eat. This accounts for only 10 percent of daily energy expenditure, and is *not* an essential factor in weight loss.

WHAT ABOUT BASAL METABOLISM?

Let's look at the first component—*basal metabolism*—which is the greatest consumer of calories, and the chief reason why dieting doesn't work. No amount of willpower can control our basal metabolism. However, basal metabolism does not remain constant. It goes up when we're ill and when we exercise. The higher our basal metabolism, the more calories we burn.

But basal metabolism can also decrease; in fact, it goes down when you diet! The reason is that when you're dieting, your body has no idea of what you're up to. It is not aware that you're trying to lose weight. Instead, the body reacts as if you're going to die!

The human animal, the product of millions of years of evolution, has survived through feast or famine. The body has survived by learning to use fuel more efficiently in times of famine; it does this by lowering its energy requirements, i.e., the basal metabolic rate. A lower basal metabolism keeps the body from starving to death until the next feast comes along—a most effective system for survival, but a dieter's nightmare.

When you cut back on calories, your body responds by immediately lowering the basal metabolic rate. And the longer the period of caloric deprivation, the greater the drop in the body's daily energy requirement. Over time, the basal metabolic rate can drop by as much as 30 percent and this change can be seen in the dieting process. When you start a diet and your basal metabolic rate is still relatively normal, it's easy to create an energy deficit. As any dieter knows, pounds come off quickly. But the longer you stay on the diet (and the longer your ignorant body continues to fight for survival), the more difficult it is to lose weight. And the longer you diet, the harder it gets. Sometimes weight loss stops entirely.

Unfortunately, the effects of a lower basal metabolism continue even after the diet ends. When you stop dieting and return to your regular eating patterns, your basal metabolism slowly returns to normal. But this recovery lags considerably behind the change in eating habits. During this lag period, weight can be gained (and frequently is) by eating the same amount of food that used to allow you to maintain your weight. Repeated going on and off diets (the yo-yo syndrome most dieters know so well) causes a cumulative lowering of the basal metabolic rate, slowing metabolic recovery even further and making weight even easier to gain! *The sad truth is, dieting is in some ways the greatest contributor to weight gain—the more you diet, the less food it takes to gain weight back.*

But the picture is even worse. The pounds you'll gain back will be in the worst possible form— pure fat. When you go on a diet, you create a caloric deficit in the body. But the body has certain nutritional requirements that it must fulfill, no matter what the caloric intake. One of these requirements is that glucose, the body's fuel, be delivered to specific parts of the body: the brain, the kidneys, and the red blood cells. While fat can eventually be used as a fuel source for the brain, it cannot be converted into glucose essential for the kidneys and red blood cells. Instead, the body must turn to another source—protein—for its glucose. And the most plentiful store of protein available to the body is muscle. What this means is that when you go on a diet, part of the weight that you lose is muscle.

When the diet fails, however, and weight is gained back, the lost muscle is not what is replenished. The regained weight comes in the form of fat. In other words, each time weight is lost and regained, the percentage of total body fat is increased. This is hardly what the dieter had in mind!

So, what about the myth "Dieting is the best way to lose weight"? The correct version is: While dieting may be a way to lose weight temporarily, in the long run it's the best way to gain weight! This doesn't mean that sustained weight loss isn't possible. But it does mean that dieting alone is not the way to do it. Read on, and you'll see how believing other myths can also keep your weight out of control.

MYTH: THERE IS (OR WILL BE) A MAGIC, PAINLESS, RAPID WAY TO LOSE WEIGHT

If only it were true! But it's not. When it comes to diet and weight control, the American public wants a miracle cure and the "diet industry" knows that a certain percentage of people will inevitably continue to jump at whatever new product comes along, perpetuating the myth, as well as the profits of the charlatans who come up with one new scheme after another.

There are two basic types of "magic weight loss" scams:

One is the "secret formula" pill that lets you eat all you want and still lose weight, even while you sleep. This "one hit" method of salesmanship (in which reorders are not a consideration) caters to consumers who want to believe anything. Look at the way the ads for these products read. Sold in quantities of 30-, 60-, or 90-day amounts, the pills are proportionately less expensive in larger quantities. The impulsive buyer will find it hard to pass up a bargain of $29.95 for 60 pills, when 30 cost $19.95 (all available to the salesman at a very low cost indeed).

The other "scam" is the one with just enough legitimacy to keep us coming back for more. These are promoted by a different brand of snake-oil salesman, a better-disguised type that I refer to as the "pseudo-scientist." The pseudo-scientist frequently has legitimate credentials, such as M.D., D.O., or Ph.D., or borrows liberally (and often incorrectly) from actual scientific research. And when these pseudo-scientists promote their miracle approaches to weight control, we assume that they know what they're talking about.

"SCIENTIFICALLY PROVEN"

A good example of this approach is the *HCG injection*. HCG (Human Chorionic Gonadotrophin) is a chemical secreted by the placenta and filtered from pregnant women's urine. The HCG injection was promoted by some medical doctors as a way to turn on special fat-burning processes in the body. Because HCG can only be given by injection, it required licensed medical personnel to administer it, and dieters to come to a clinic regularly. It had all the appearances of a serious cure. The only problem was that the product didn't work, and had absolutely no scientific basis. What it did have was a strong placebo effect, due largely to the commitment involved on the part of the dieters. But that's all.

Another more recent example of this can be seen in the use of daily or weekly *vitamin B-12 shots,* which are said to augment weight loss. Despite the fact that there is no scientific evidence to support this claim whatsoever, these injections continue to be promoted, and believed in, as a cure for obesity.

Even legitimate scientific research can feed into the myth of the miracle cure when falsely applied or misinterpreted. Take *tryptophan,* for example. Tryptophan is an amino acid that the body converts into a chemical called serotonin. Serotonin is a very hot topic in obesity research today. We are exploring the role it plays in making us feel hungry or full and satisfied. Serotonin, which aids the brain in transmitting messages from one nerve cell to another, seems to play a particularly important role in sending messages to the group of cells concerned with the subjective experiences of hunger and satiety. Overeating may indicate that a lower level of serotonin is reaching these cells, and one solution to this problem might be to increase the serotonin supply.

Consequently, delivering more tryptophan to the brain (either with tryptophan pills or through tryptophan-rich foods) could help to raise the level of serotonin and aid in weight control. Another approach might be the use of drugs that increase the amount of serotonin in the brain.

This sounds like the miracle cure that we've all been waiting for. However, if we listen more carefully, we will learn that taking a few grams of tryptophan does not necessarily mean what we think it will. The serotonin research being conducted relates only to a small percentage of compulsive overeaters with weight problems. And at best, for this minority, increasing brain serotonin might be a partial solution to their problems (this research is still in progress). But numerous other factors that are also important in weight regulation must be considered along with this discovery. And medical scientists working on serotonin research do not see it as a miracle cure for weight control.

The biological system that determines weight control, and all the behavioral, emotional, psychological, and cultural influences that go along with it, is extremely complex. And the likelihood of coming up with a simple, single solution is minimal. What legitimate scientific research confirms is that partial solutions will be uncovered—solutions that will help some people and not others.

MYTH: "YOU CAN LOSE TEN POUNDS OF UGLY FAT IN SEVEN DAYS"

Now this sounds familiar! And it's hard to resist. We all want to "quick start" and get a diet going, and quick success inspires you to keep at it. It's only natural, and the diet entrepreneurs know it too. Actually it is physically impossible to lose ten pounds of real weight in seven days by dieting alone.

The three basic food types are fats, proteins, and carbohydrates. Historically, of these three major food groups, we have blamed carbohydrates as the primary culprits for causing weight gain. For many years low-carbohydrate/high-protein diets, and even low-carbohydrate/high-fat diets, have been in vogue. While it is possible to shed ten pounds on a low-carbohydrate diet, the pounds lost are mainly water—probably not the ten pounds of fat you had in mind when you began the diet.

The reason you lose weight in such a short time on a low-carbohydrate diet is quite simple. Seventy percent of your body weight is water. Most of it is stored within the cells (intracellular water), and a smaller fraction is in the blood (extra cellular water). These two water compartments normally coexist in a friendly equilibrium, each borrowing from the other when needed, such as when the blood needs extra water from the cells to help wash out toxins (or poisons) from the body. A low-carbohydrate diet actually *produces* toxins, resulting in the cells' water being released into the blood system to help wash away the toxins.

Low-carbohydrate diets produce toxins because the body, without its usual supply of carbohydrates, is forced to rely on proteins and fats for its fuel. Ketones (toxins from fat) and nitrogen (toxins from protein) are produced. Because they cannot be allowed to accumulate in the body, they're flushed out with water (especially early in the diet, when the body has not fully adjusted to the ketones).

As a result, during the beginning stage of a diet, you lose a good amount of water. And that can be a lot of pounds (try picking up a gallon of juice with one hand to find out). Your scale does not distinguish between fat and water loss. So what seems like great progress is really water loss and will soon be gained back.

And what about the fat? I say again, it simply isn't possible to lose ten pounds of fat in seven days. Here's some more basic physiology. Did you know that body fat can be measured in calories? One pound of body fat equals 3,500 calories. To lose a pound of fat, you must expend 3,500 more calories than you consume.

This may not sound too difficult, until you realize that the usual amount of energy expended by a person runs from 1,500 to 3,000 calories a day. Even if you fast for 24 hours, the average person, following a normal daily routine, still would not lose one pound of fat.

When you go on a diet, you do cut back on caloric intake, but, as you've probably already guessed, you can't possibly create a 35,000 calorie deficit (the amount necessary to lose ten pounds of fat) in only one week, even if you eat absolutely nothing!

What these quick-weight-loss schemes are in fact relying on is the body's loss of water. And beyond that, the truth is that when you reintroduce carbohydrates into your diet (usually when you're sick and tired of not having them anymore), something devastating happens. The old water equilibrium is immediately reestablished, and you regain the lost weight as rapidly as you lost it initially. Anyone who has experienced the inexplicable "I go off my diet for one day and gain six pounds!" knows this experience all too well.

So, don't set yourself up for inevitable disappointment by buying into the concept of the quick-weight-loss program. The only thing you'll lose is your money.

MYTH: IF YOU WANT TO CONTROL YOUR WEIGHT, THERE ARE SOME FOODS YOU SHOULD NEVER EAT ("FORBIDDEN FOODS")

This myth derives largely from beliefs about the dangers of carbohydrates, and from the false assumption that the dieter *must* always avoid certain "diet-killing" foods, such as ice cream, pizza, and Twinkies.

The notion that carbohydrates (such as bread and pasta) should be avoided is largely based on the low-carbohydrate diets that were popular years ago. Nutritionists have repeatedly dismissed these diets as unsound. It was believed that the less carbohydrates we eat, the more rapid our weight loss will be. As we've already discussed (see page 20), what low-carbohydrate diets induce is rapid water loss. The facts are, that when it comes to lasting weight control, low-carbohydrate diets are senseless, and sometimes downright dangerous.

The truth is that carbohydrates themselves aren't all that bad. In fact, the worst food culprit isn't carbohydrates at all, it's *fat*.

Here are the facts. There are three food classes—protein, carbohydrates, and fat. Each has its own particular caloric density (calories per unit weight). Proteins and carbohydrates have equal caloric density, each containing 4.5 calories per gram. Fat, on the other hand, has 9 calories per gram. That's right. Every bite of fat has twice the calories of a bite of protein or carbohydrates. Additionally, fat (especially in the saturated form found in animal fat) may cause other significant health problems, such as hypertension and heart disease. If any food class were to be forbidden, it would have to be fat. (But even this isn't sensible or nutritionally sound. Ingested fat plays an important role in the body, too. It's just that Americans tend to consume too high a percentage of it on a daily basis.)

Carbohydrates actually are excellent weight control foods, especially complex carbohydrates (such as those found in pasta, whole-grain bread, and vegetable fiber). They take longer to digest than other foods and break down into glucose (the final product in the carbohydrate metabolism). As a result, they may enhance and prolong our sense of fullness and satisfaction. Complex carbohydrates may also aid in weight control by allowing for a smooth rise and fall in plasma insulin, something which may help to control hunger.

And what about other forbidden foods—pizza, ice cream, candy, bacon, etc.? First of all, these are obviously not all carbohydrates (there's a lot of fat in pizza). But can you control your weight and still eat these foods? Surely it would help us stay thin if we could just forget about these foods forever.

Let's do some analyzing of the diet mentality. Dieting is not a normal state of affairs, and chronic dieting is not a normal way of life (although it certainly is common). The constant deprivation, mental dialogue, guilt, and fear begin to work on the dieter, to the point that losing weight and sticking to a diet begin to become life-defining imperatives. According to the diet mentality, sticking to your diet, or blowing it, labels you as a good or a bad person. Resisting forbidden food is good; giving in is a sin. Food becomes a highly emotional issue, and research has shown that clinging to the concept of "forbidden foods" guarantees a binge on those foods, as soon as the diet is broken. And let's be honest, any diet that forbids any foods is eventually broken.

The problem with foods like pizza, ice cream, and candy is their caloric density. These foods do have a lot of calories per bite, and to really control your weight, you must eat all calorically dense food in moderation. And, beware: Many foods that have been traditionally considered good diet foods—cottage cheese, for example—are also calorically dense.

If you want to develop a healthy eating style and long-term weight control you must learn which foods are calorically dense. Package labeling can really help here; check the number of calories per serving and the number of servings in the package.

"FORBIDDEN" FOODS vs. "GOOD" FOODS

Take a look at the following lists of common foods. Most people would consider the foods in the first column to be "forbidden" foods (or foods to be avoided) and the foods in the second column to be "good" foods. However, as the calorie totals indicate, the "forbidden" and "good" labels can be very misleading. In fact, these so-called "forbidden" foods are actually no worse than their "good" food counterparts.

"Forbidden" Foods	calories	"Good" Foods	calories
Sour cream (1 tbsp.)	25	Yogurt (flavored) 8 ounce cup	240
Bread (1 slice)	60	Cottage cheese (1 cup)	200
Pasta (8 ounces)	200	Tuna salad (1 cup)	400
Pizza (1 slice)	250	Lean ground beef (¼ lb. cooked)	350
Chocolate bar	240	Salad with 2 tbsp. of dressing	240

MYTH: IT'S BEST TO WEIGH YOURSELF
EVERY DAY

At The Sharper Image, the prestigious mail order catalog store, you can buy a scale that talks.
Too bad it isn't programmed to say what most dieters are longing to hear—"You've lost two
pounds. You're just terrific. Now you're going to
have a great day!" Every morning when we step
onto the scale, hoping against hope that it's down,
we're ready to hear that speech. But more often,
we see what we feared most—no loss or, even
worse, weight gain.

Weighing ourselves every day is a setup for disaster! The scale is hardly a neutral object in the
dieter's life. And we're not just talking about once
a day. Many people go for a progress report three,
four, or five times daily, eagerly willing to measure success even by the quarter pound.

The scale is dangerous. The abuse of water pills
and laxatives can easily be justified when losing
pounds at any cost becomes the central goal. Fortunately science has something to tell us when it
comes to scale-watching—the scale can have a distinct purpose, but only when it is used in a way
that truly monitors the changes in our bodies.

To decide how often it makes sense to weigh
yourself, let's look at the time frame in which various body weight components change. Basic phys-

iology tells us that some components of the body—such as bones, skin, and organs—change weight very slowly during development, and once growth is completed, stop changing weight. Muscle tissue can change weight during adulthood; however, the time frame for measuring changes in muscle weight takes about a month. As we know, body fat can also change weight. Remembering the basic fact that a pound of fat equals 3,500 calories and that creating a deficit or excess of 3,500 calories takes some time—usually three to four days—the shortest time frame that will show a legitimate change in body fat is about a week.

How is it possible, then, that some people do lose 2 or 3 pounds in a day? Easy. Remember our old friend water weight? Water weight can change quite rapidly, and is the *only* body component that changes on a daily basis. But as we know, losing water weight isn't losing body fat. In a way, it's a false weight loss and can completely overshadow the one-quarter pound of body fat that may be lost in a day of a reasonable diet. So, *weigh yourself once a week at most; less frequently is even better.* You'll eliminate some of the senseless anxiety that comes from constant scale watching. And you'll be seeing how your body gains or loses fat, not water.

MYTH: **EXERCISE IS AN OPTIONAL COMPONENT OF A WEIGHT CONTROL PROGRAM; IT'S THE DIET THAT COUNTS**

Pick up any best-selling diet book, and the chances are pretty good there will be little mention of exercise. Certainly, it won't be the focus of the book. Exercise isn't a popular recommendation. Studies have shown that people are much more willing to embark on a new diet than they are to begin an exercise program. And since authors of diet books are in the business of selling books, they're far more likely to give you something they think you'll want, something along the lines of the previously discussed miracle cure. I believe, however, a regular exercise program *must* be a part of any weight control effort.

Let's examine why exercise must be an integral part of our normal daily routine. In looking at the role that physical exercise can play for us, we should consider some basic physiology and recent scientific research.

The following energy equation, first discussed on page 12, can help us here.

**Energy Consumed − Energy Expended =
Body Fat (Gained or Lost)**

Remember, body fat loss occurs when Energy Expended exceeds Energy Consumed (food). For simplicity's sake, we'll say that Energy Expended is equal to approximately two-thirds basal metabolic rate (remember, the basal metabolic rate refers to the amount of energy your body needs to keep your heart beating, lungs working, etc.) and one-third physical activity. First, we'll focus on the physical activity component.

The facts are simple. Physical activity burns calories: The more physical activity, the greater the caloric deficit. The number of calories a particular activity requires depends on a number of factors, including the rigorousness of the activity, genetic factors, body weight, and duration. We've all seen those calorie tables that tell us that a very vigorous activity, like running six miles in an hour, can burn well over 600 calories, while a game of tennis can burn about 400. These numbers can frequently be discouraging when compared to the calorie content of some of our favorite foods. (To burn off a Big Mac, fries, and a Coke, you'll have to run for about two hours.) From this viewpoint, it's easy to see why dieting appears easier than losing weight by exercising; driving past McDonald's is a lot less tiring than enduring a two-hour run. If exercise were no more than a calorie tradeoff, then it might make sense, but that's vastly undervaluing its function.

The human body was designed to be more physically active than we are today. Increasing physical activity makes the whole system work better. A sense of fitness and well-being is rewarding in and of itself. And research is suggesting that the rewarding feeling may actually be part of a biochemical process, not simply a psychological effect. It appears that physical exercise induces the brain to release chemicals called endorphins (an internal, natural painkiller), giving the exerciser a sense of well-being and comfort. Exercise also often tends to lessen, rather than increase appetite, helping to keep caloric intake down. These factors alone might be reason enough to make exercise a part of your life. But beyond this, exercise can raise the basal metabolic rate, and that's great.

If you remember, the basal metabolic rate is our greatest consumer of calories. As caloric intake goes down, so does the basal metabolic rate. When trying to lose weight, exercise, especially regular exercise, can help to restore the basal metabolic rate to pre-dieting levels.

Additionally, research shows that a specific type, duration, and intensity of exercise is necessary to achieve this desired effect. The best way to bring up the basal metabolic rate is with aerobic exercise—physical activity that increases the heart and breathing rates. Aerobic exercise includes activities such as vigorous walking, running, bicycling, basketball, tennis, and raquetball; and of course, plain old aerobics. It does not include weight lifting and Nautilus training (these are anaerobic exercises designed to strengthen and build muscles). All of the aerobic exercises will raise the pulse to the point necessary to affect the basal metabolism. It's also been found that aerobic exercise will result in maximum benefit if done in thirty-minute sessions four times a week. As you can see, exercise is the most important part of any weight control program. While fad diet books ignore it, anyone who is getting smart about weight control can't afford to!

MYTH: IT'S POSSIBLE TO SPOT REDUCE

"Okay, today we're going to work on the hips and thighs." That's the kind of thing you're likely to hear when you turn on an exercise program on TV. Following this introduction, the instructor will usually present a series of exercises specifically designed to attack those problem areas and get them back into proportion with the rest of the body. The exercises look right, and when you do them, it certainly feels like you're fixing what you want to fix. But are you? The answer is no.

While exercising a specific area of your body may do wonders for the underlying muscle, the layers of fat above will still remain. Therefore, any attempts to "spot reduce," such as trying to eliminate a flabby midsection, will fail—unless of course the "spot reduction" is accompanied by an overall, effective exercise and weight control program. Why will a spot reduction program by itself fail?

To begin with, exercising a particular "spot" on your body won't result in burning off fat in that area. The body determines its energy requirements as a whole, not in parts. Whether the burning of calories comes from jogging, pull-ups, housework, or sex, it's all the same to the body. A calorie burned is a calorie burned, and fat deposits are usually called upon uniformly to give up their energy when there is a need. So, once again, the ignorant body is unaware; it doesn't know that when you do 100 leg lifts you're trying to lose fat on your legs, not on your arms or face.

This doesn't mean that spot exercising does nothing for the area being exercised. Selective exercise can tone, strengthen, and even enlarge muscle mass in a particular area. The muscle, however, remains below the deposit of fat. And because exercise will only tone or strengthen muscles, not the connective tissue or the fat above them, unless total body fat is reduced, toning and strengthening the muscle will not in itself create a lean, defined line or shape.

Any discussion of spot reducing must at least touch on the latest rage in an already crowded arena of products and techniques—*liposuction*. Liposuction (the physical removal of fat deposits by surgical procedure) is clearly the hottest thing in plastic surgery today. It's quick, and it requires no dieting or exercise (except what it takes to remove your wallet from your pocket).

But is this the way to go? Let's look at the risks involved versus the benefits. The risks include those generally associated with surgery and the use of anesthesia, or at the very least, significant subjective disappointment with the outcome. The benefits include removal of stubborn fat deposits that you may not be able to get rid of any other way. Generally there are satisfactory results, and relatively low risk when performed by an experienced and reliable plastic surgeon. The choice is not to be made lightly; however, if you want to spend the money, and you've assessed the risk/benefit ratio and feel it's something you're willing to chance, then, yes, it may be possible to "spot" reduce surgically. This is an important decision that should *only* be made in consultation with a highly qualified and experienced physician.

MYTH: IT'S BETTER TO START EXERCISING AFTER YOU LOSE WEIGHT; IT'S EASIER AND SAFER

How many times have you heard, "I'll start exercising as soon as I take off a few pounds"? This is a common concern, involving worry about ease and safety, and, to be honest, also a good dose of anxiety about appearance. However, these concerns are not warranted.

The fact is, contrary to what many people think, it is *not* easier for a thinner person to get into shape. A thinner person may have an easier time with a flight of stairs, but this doesn't mean that he or she's in shape. Put most thin people and an overweight person on stationary bicycles, both working against the same level of resistance of the machine, and you'll find little difference in terms of endurance or pain. *That's because it's difficult for all people to get in shape, regardless of their size.* Getting in shape requires a graduated and sustained effort, and a commitment to regular participation. So the excuse of "I'm waiting until I lose some weight first" really doesn't make sense, and is in fact only delaying the benefits that exercise provides in any effective weight control program.

What about safety? Does additional weight actually create greater risk for the exerciser? Let's first examine this from a life-and-death viewpoint. Aerobic exercise can cause death, if it's putting a strain on an already weak heart. The extra strain of exercise can reveal underlying heart disease that might not have previously been detected. *That's why people in their mid-30s or older should consult a physician for cardiovascular testing before beginning an exercise program. It's not body fat that endangers the exerciser, it's a bad heart!*

What about injuries? Here, there are some special considerations to take into account. It's true, the heavier you are, the more likely it is that certain exercises may cause injuries. Again, thin people can get injured, too, but it's just common sense that a heavier person will put more strain on joints and muscles when exercising than a thinner person. But this is not a legitimate excuse for the heavier person. If anything, there are now more cardiovascular fitness machines that allow you to work against the resistance of the machine rather than against your own body weight.

And finally, there's the issue of vanity. Health clubs look great and are the perfect place to get started on an aerobic training program. But let's face it. Along with all the equipment, able instructors, and encouraging atmosphere, is something else—those dreaded exercise outfits! And there seems to be an endless parade of people who look like they're in good shape and look even better in a leotard. The vanity issue may be hard to acknowledge, and certainly can be difficult to overcome. But since any successful weight control program must include exercise, you're going to have to deal with it. Go with a friend, but do it! And once you're there, try looking around. You may find that everyone doesn't look as terrific as you first thought. Maybe there just happened to be a few more noticeable ones who caught your eye. Try looking at the others around you as critically as you do yourself, and you'll begin to see that practically everyone's got some bulges to contend with. Don't put off exercising until you lose some weight. As you'll see in chapter 6, the only thing that makes sense is to start exercising first. Weight loss will definitely follow.

MYTH: YOU CAN'T EXERCISE TOO MUCH

This myth is like the old saying "You can't be too rich or too thin." It sounds good, but it can cause trouble.

Over the past decade, fitness has graduated from being a "hobby" for some to a craze pursued by millions. Unfortunately, some exercisers have gravitated to "workouts" with the same vengeance and obsession as others might use to follow an extreme diet. Our purpose is to explode myths about weight control, so that you can take an approach that is sensible, rational, and realistic. This also applies when it comes to physical exercise.

There's a new syndrome being discussed in the medical journals—the plight of the *obligate exerciser*. This is a person who begins to develop a mind-set about exercising and fitness not unlike that of an anorexic in regard to food and weight control. For the obligate exerciser, and for many who may not be quite this extreme but who have become overly invested emotionally in exercise, physical activity is not simply a component of a more natural, healthier life-style, but rather an end in itself. For this group, exercise can be a preoccupation that actually detracts from its benefits.

The obligate exerciser begins to fear missing an exercise session in the same way the chronic dieter fears breaking a diet. Deviation spells disaster.

Anxiety about exercise—the inner compulsion to go further, do more, get the "burn," go to the class more often—becomes the mental focus. While TV and magazines might make this approach seem healthy, the fact is that it's not. Intensive aerobics, Nautilus machines, and free weights on a daily basis are not what the body was designed for, and what may have begun as an attempt to reach a more "natural" condition can be far from it. On both the emotional and physical level, this type of extreme behavior can be damaging.

The field of sports medicine has developed as an answer to the needs of exercise-conscious Americans. This has been a godsend for the professional athlete. But the fact is that the sports medicine specialist spends most of his or her day patching up the "obligate" fitness fanatics. The number of muscle and bone problems emerging from the fitness craze is ever-growing. More than one orthopedist has gone on record criticizing jogging as causing extreme strain on the legs. And this is only one of the many physical ailments that are showing up as a result of compulsive exercise. The new and growing practice of using steroids to speed muscle growth is insanely dangerous.

Remember that even a good exercise program can become a dangerous obsession. The old adage still applies—doing everything in moderation is the best and healthiest approach.

-------------- **CHAPTER** --------------
3

The Biological Myths

MYTH: OBESITY IS A DISEASE

Obesity is not a disease. We know for certain that
body fat is human tissue that exists in varying
amounts in various people. Some people have ill-
nesses that are worsened by excess body fat, and
they should try to reduce their weight. But beyond
that, the concept of obesity as a disease is probably
doing more psychological harm than physical good.

You may be surprised to know that even in obesity research, there's a lot of controversy about the
issue of who should be labeled "obese." One re-
searcher was heard to say that if people are not
too fat, you should refer to them as "overweight"
so as not to hurt their feelings, and if they're extremely fat, then you can call them "obese." It is
also common to refer to people who are 100 percent (or by some definitions 100 pounds) overweight as "morbidly obese"; this arbitrary cutoff
has important implications for insurance coverage
on certain surgical procedures. Why can't the ex-

perts agree on a definition of who's obese and who isn't? It seems simple enough, but in fact it's not simple at all.

Many human attributes are statistically defined—either you have them or you don't, like blue eyes or blond hair. It is also true for most diseases; there may be variations in terms of severity, but it's usually easy to define the people who do or do not have a particular disease. But what about obesity?

Body weight is distributed on a continuum, in the pattern of a bell-shaped curve. If you take everyone's body weight and put it on a graph, placing the number of pounds on the horizontal axis and the number of people on the vertical axis, you'll find the common statistical outcome. It looks like this:

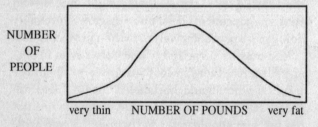

NUMBER
OF
PEOPLE

very thin   NUMBER OF POUNDS   very fat

Most people's weight clusters around the middle, with fewer and fewer the closer you get to the very fat or very thin extremes. But if obesity is something that can be defined, then some people must have it while others do not. To prove this, it would be necessary to draw a line on the graph and pronounce that everyone above that line has the disease and everyone below it doesn't. Picture the bell curve as an IQ scale. Draw a line at the middle—say, 120 on the IQ scale. Everyone above the line is smart while those below it are not. This just doesn't make sense. The point here is that any definition of obesity is arbitrary. And since the majority of people who consider themselves to be overweight are in the middle of the bell-shaped curve (only 1 percent of the overweight population is "morbidly obese"), any such definition involves labeling a large group of people "sick." This has some extreme implications for both the self-esteem and pursuit of weight loss for a considerable portion of the population.

What about the insurance tables of ideal body weights? If you're above the weight levels listed on those charts, doesn't it mean you're overweight? In common practice, this is the standard used. For now, let's just say that if we accept the insurance table guidelines, all we have is another way of labeling some people with the "disease" of obesity.

A definition of obesity might be helpful if we were diagnosing a condition with a predictable or expected negative outcome that could be treated. But in the case of "excess" body weight, or more precisely, "excess" body fat, it's not at all clear that we're dealing with a condition that has a defined or predictable negative outcome.

We know that obesity itself does not act like a disease; it does not kill people, debilitate them, or even make them sick. It is simply an arbitrary definition, based on the amount of a particular tissue in the body. From this viewpoint, it's no different from being taller than other people. And taller people are not referred to as "sick," or "overheight." The question is whether "excess" body fat causes damage to other parts of the body that then can kill people or impair their health. The answer to this is probably yes, but only in some people. And those are people who have a medical condition that is worsened by excessive body weight and will improve by losing weight. This does not mean that obesity is the disease. What it's in fact saying is that losing weight may be a medicine for other diseases.

Disease is a negative and frightening concept, and should not be referred to lightly. Calling obesity a disease is thoughtless. There is no actual definition of this condition, and it does not behave like a disease. In a culture obsessed with thinness, this kind of labeling is destructive. Most people who are above the ideal body weight levels are only mildly or moderately so. To classify an entire, usually healthy group of our society as "diseased" is neither justified nor useful.

MYTH: IT'S NORMAL TO BE THIN

It's not normal to be thin—it's normal to be you.
How many times have you heard: "There's a thin person within everyone, just waiting to get out."

Or, "The way to make a fat person a thin person is to get them to think and act like a thin person."

These are the kinds of widely held prejudices that are commonly heard in our society. Years ago researchers believed the had found clear-cut differences between the eating behavior and activity levels of obese people and thin people. And through behavioral techniques, they tried to train obese people to become "thin people."

These techniques are still reflected in various forms in diet programs today. "Put down your fork between each bite" is a frequent recommendation. The premise here is that people who wolf down their food become fat, whereas thin people savor each mouthful. This may sound like it makes sense, but it doesn't. Numerous studies have shown that no predictable set of eating behaviors or activity levels exists to differentiate fat people from thin people. Some thin people wolf down their food. The overweight person with this particular eating style may well benefit from following the advice to eat more slowly, but in universal terms it is simply not applicable.

Another commonly held belief is that people become fat because they're more highly responsive to the taste and palatability of food, and less responsive to inner hunger and satiety feelings. This concept is known as the externality theory, and was widely accepted at one time. Fat people are often stereotyped as not being able to control themselves around food (like the fat people depicted in TV shows). Again, this theory may sound attractive, but it's just not true. Many people—fat, thin, and normal—can't resist tempting food and respond more strongly to external than to internal cues when they eat.

Is a lean body the most natural and healthful way to be for everyone? In a world in which we are very concerned with the numerous destructive and polluting forces ruining our environment and our bodies, we are bent on seeking the most natural and healthy path. But does this necessarily translate into the body being naturally thin? Do we truly "fight" nature by gaining weight? In fact, the opposite may be the case. Let's look at one of the most intriguing theories now being developed in obesity research—the setpoint theory of body weight regulation.

In a way, our minds are at war with our bodies. An examination of the *setpoint theory* begins to make this all the more clear.

Picture your home thermostat. When you set the temperature to 72 degrees, it does not go above or below that point; when the temperature gets too low, the thermostat compensates for the deviation by turning on the furnace; and when it reaches the desired temperature again, it turns the furnace off. This is a simple setpoint mechanism. Many obesity researchers believe that body fat is regulated on a setpoint basis as well. The mechanism, however, is not nearly as simple as that of the thermostat, nor is it as fully understood.

Our bodies seem to be most comfortable with a certain percentage of body fat, and in fact go to great lengths to protect that balance. Substantial research, based on human and animal studies, points to the fact that the body seems to have its own ability to regulate and maintain a certain percentage of fat, calling compensatory mechanisms into play when total fat deviates from the desired level. As we have already noted, when someone attempts to diet to a point below their setpoint of fat, the metabolism slows down to compensate. There are also other mechanisms that function to maintain this setpoint. Enzymes that regulate fat deposition may be involved. And there are specific centers in the brain that regulate hunger and appetite, undoubtedly playing an important part in monitoring the setpoint and responding to deviations. There are still many aspects of the setpoint theory of body fat to be uncovered, but it does present a new twist when considering the body weight issue. No longer can "thin" be strictly equated with "normal."

So, what determines an individual's setpoint? What decides the amount of body fat any one person is "meant" to have? Certainly genetics plays a central role; the tendency to deposit fat is at least in part something that is passed down from parent to child. There are also environmental and behavior factors at work in determining the setpoint. Prolonged periods of excessive eating or significant slowing down of physical activity may raise the setpoint. So can physiological events such as pregnancy. Something else that typically raises the setpoint is the elimination of nicotine from the body. When people stop smoking, it characteristically shifts their setpoint upward by about ten pounds. While this is often attributed to an increase in eating to compensate for the oral loss of cigarettes, the effect seems to be a long-term weight shift—the establishment of a new setpoint or stable weight that is very hard to change.

Setting a weight that resists change is what the setpoint mechanism seems to do. This is not actually a single point, but rather a range of weight, below which (and sometimes above which) it's difficult to move. Anyone who has tried to control weight knows it's easy to lose pounds in the beginning, but over time it becomes harder and harder, or even impossible. You have approached your setpoint. At some time, you may have actually managed to reach a target weight that was well below your setpoint, and in looking back, you will probably recall that it was nearly impossible to maintain that weight. That's because you were fighting nature—or trying to get your body to be at an unnatural, abnormal weight for you! What's normal and natural for each person is to be at their setpoint weight, which is not necessarily thin. But don't give up hope too quickly because the good news is that it is possible to lower your setpoint with exercise. And it's also true that there are any people whose weight is well above their setpoint due to chronic overeating. But science is clearly telling us it's not "normal" for everyone to be thin; it's more normal for everyone to be at their setpoint weight.

**MYTH: FAT PARENTS HAVE FAT
         CHILDREN BECAUSE THEY
         TEACH THEM BAD EATING
         HABITS**

   This is not the simple answer as to why there are fat families. There are a combination of factors at work here. What our parents teach us (nurture) is important, but what we inherit from our parents biologically (nature) may be even more crucial in determining our weight.

   Statistical studies show that children of overweight parents are at substantially higher risk of becoming overweight adults themselves. Some studies put this figure as high as 80 percent. But is this entirely due to what parents teach their children or is it biologically determined? This issue is at the forefront of obesity research today.

   Let's examine some of the theories now being explored.

   NURTURE
   Can you teach someone to be fat? Many people believe that this is true. If a home environment encourages overeating, it makes sense that deeply ingrained patterns of overeating behavior will be

formed and taken from childhood into adult life. Eating in response to stress, for example, or rewarding yourself with food, are habits that are learned and encouraged at an early age. And when calorically rich food is overused, the outcome seems inevitable. Studies also tell us that the more hours a child spends in front of the television, the more likely it is that he or she will become obese. The parent's guidance has a lot to do with how much TV a child watches, and perhaps more importantly, with how much food the child eats while watching. Many over-weight adults can look back at childhoods in which they were taught to overeat and eat for the wrong reasons. These habits are difficult to break, and many of the life-style changes promoted in weight control programs are directed at correcting these deeply ingrained patterns of behavior. "When you've accomplished a difficult task, don't reward yourself with a sundae. Try a nice walk in the sunshine, or a warm bath." But does a walk compare with a sundae? Old habits are not easy to change.

An environmental theory of obesity does make sense, and correcting poor eating habits can go a long way in helping to control weight. But look around. Not everyone who eats a lot is obese. And the reverse is also true—not all overweight people overeat. Obesity researchers are now paying closer attention to this reality, and they're coming up with some interesting findings about what nature biologically determines about body weight.

NATURE

If there's one area of medical research that holds promise for miraculous advances in health care, it's genetics. Some of our worst diseases are genetically based, and with the efforts now going on in genetic research, it may become possible to alter and correct genetic defects. Genetics also plays a significant role in determining body weight. But before we explore that, let's look briefly at how genes work.

Genes are collections of DNA, the chemical that guides the creation of all the cells in the body. We are all born with a specific set of genes as a result of certain combinations we inherit from our parents. The simplest type of gene transference from parent to child is when a single gene or pair of genes causes a single trait.

There are some instances of obesity that are transmitted by a single genetic defect, but these conditions are very rare, and they are also accompanied by additional physical problems. According to obesity researchers, the tendency to accumulate excess body fat in otherwise normal people is not controlled by a single gene. The biological side of weight regulation is polygenetic—it is influenced by many biological factors, and each of those is controlled by one or more genes. How have the scientists figured this out? It's complicated, and in some ways what they're doing is starting at the finish line and working backward.

The "finish," or outcome, of the combined genetic influences is the total amount of fat in the adult body. Dr. Albert Stunkard's study,* "An Adoption Study of Human Obesity," firmly established that genetically based biological factors figure strongly in determining what the total body fat will be. Dr. Stunkard took a large group of adults, all of whom were adopted as children. He wanted to determine if the body weight of an adult who had been an adopted child (someone not brought up by his or her biological parents) would resemble the adoptive parents or the biological parents. If the child resembled the adoptive parents, then the environment must be the stronger influence; and if the child resembled the biological parents, then genetics must be the more powerful force. The results of this study were overwhelmingly conclusive. Genetics factors were of much greater influence than the environment. With this known, the next big question became, how does this happen? And the "how" is what genetic obesity research is all about.

What the researchers are now investigating is exactly what the biological differences are that determine body weight. And they're coming up with new information constantly. For a start, let's look briefly at a few of the findings.

Keep in mind the old energy equation we now

*Stunkard, A.J., Thorkild, I.A., Sorensen, et al. "An Adoption Study of Human Obesity," *New England Journal of Medicine.* vol. 314, no. 4 (1986), pp. 193–198.

know so well—Body Fat is equal to Energy Consumed minus Energy Expended. Researchers are now discovering that there are biological mechanisms that influence body weight at all points of this equation. Let's start with "excess energy." Excess energy is characteristically stored as body fat. But while this may be the general rule, excess energy is not always stored as fat in all people. Some people do not store excess energy at all, but simply burn it off harmlessly as heat in a process called dietary induced thermogenesis (DIT). It is not yet a proven fact, but there is a good amount of evidence pointing to the possibility that some people are genetically protected from being overweight by active DIT mechanism. We all know thin people who eat like horses (you know one, don't you?) and never gain weight.

Now, let's turn to the "Energy Consumed" part of the equation. Is the amount and type of food we eat determined solely by what we learn, or are genetic factors at work here too? A conference on obesity at the New York Academy of Sciences recently explored this question in depth. What's emerging is that there indeed may be genetically caused biological forces that drive some people to consume more calories than others, with a particular urge toward carbohydrates. This may at least partially help to explain the so-called compulsive eater (we'll explore this later).

Finally, there's "Energy Expenditure." We know that genetics determine different basal (resting) metabolic rates and different rates of metabolic response to physical exercise in different people. The same caloric intake that might have little or no effect on the weight of someone with a higher basal metabolic rate, can result in weight gain for a person with a lower rate. Some people are simply more efficient machines than others; they require less fuel to run the body, and this means that they must eat less than others to control their weight.

This is by no means a complete list of all the possible genetic factors that play into body weight. But we can see the general trend—nature is crucial to our weight regulation patterns. Let's step back and look again at what we've just seen. Genetics and environment both significantly affect body weight. In a famine, everyone—obese and skinny alike—would be thin (although the obese would live longer due to greater efficiency in calorie utilization). In an environment where calorically rich food is readily available, however, and where early learning has led to habits of overeating, someone with a genetic makeup that tends toward overweight will turn out to be obese. There is a dynamic interplay between the environmental and biological forces at work when it comes to body weight regulation and we know now that simply changing eating behavior will not affect all of the factors that determine body weight.

MYTH: DIETING CAN'T HURT

Dieting can be hurtful and dangerous. It can cause weight gain and an increase in body fat. It can have dangerous physical effects on your body. And repeated dieting can cause obsessional behavior that puts you at risk for abusing pills, laxatives, diuretics, and can lead to conditions such as bulimia. Put simply, dieting can be a serious hazard to your health.

In our society, it's hard not to diet. And even if someone were to reasonably argue to the contrary, you would probably say, "Well, certainly it can't hurt." And why should you think otherwise? You keep reading about how being overweight is bad for your health; they say it takes years off your life; and your friends, family, and doctor all keep mentioning that you could stand to lose a few pounds. Nobody ever seems to tell you that cutting back on your calories could possibly be bad for you. But it can be.

We know that repetitive on-and-off dieting has a cumulative effect on the body that slows down the metabolic rate. When you begin to eat normally again, you find that the same food that once allowed you to maintain your weight now makes you gain—the results of your lower basal metabolic rate. And when you begin to replace the muscle tissue lost in the diet, it comes back in the form of fat and you're stuck with a higher body fat content than before. These risks are highest on fad diets, very low-calorie diets, and low-carbohydrate diets. But even a sensible, nutritionally balanced diet causes a lowered metabolic response. But this is only the beginning of the problem.

A study conducted during World War II showed exactly how starvation affects human beings. In this experiment, which involved putting a group of young men on a 1,700-calorie-a-day diet for six months, the caloric deprivation was similar to that which dieters experience. At the beginning of the experiment, there was a brief period in which the young men experienced increased energy and mild euphoria (not unlike that which many dieters feel). And then came the characteristic symptoms of caloric deprivation—ceaseless hunger, irritability, anger, preoccupation with food, and lethargy. These symptoms grew worse over the six months. By the end of the experiment, the young men were in frightening condition. Once off the diet, they gorged themselves until they gained back all the lost weight. And it took up to nine months for a feeling of normality to be restored.

The body is simply not geared to accept prolonged calorie deprivation, and it will do everything in its power to fight against it—to get past the famine. Extreme diets can cause personal suffering, suffering at work, and suffering on the part of your family who must live through the physical and emotional effects the diet has on you. Is that what you want from your diet?

There are also notable hormonal imbalances associated with dieting. It's well known that female anorexics stop having their menstrual cycle. That's because body fat is crucial to the female hormonal system. Dieting also often disrupts the regularity of the menstrual cycle by causing hormonal imbalances. Listen to your body when it responds unnaturally to what is supposedly a health-promoting activity! You're not making yourself healthier; you're hurting your natural balance.

When you think about the obsession involved in dieting combined with the physiological changes it causes, dieting can lead to dangerous eating behaviors like binging and purging.

Caloric deprivation by definition causes intense hunger and preoccupation with food. That's what the brain dictates. Then, there's the forbidden food factor, with the loss of favorite foods furthering the sense of deprivation. And add to that, the diet cycle mentality—what it means to be on or off your diet. All of this creates the perfect setup for binging. If you've denied yourself cookies, ice cream, pizza, and pastrami sandwiches for long enough, you're going to want to eat each one of them again before you start on the next diet. Some binges are intense and short-lived, while others are prolonged and only end when all the weight is gained back. (This is common.) But the pervasiveness of the diet-binge-diet pattern is unquestionable.

Dieting followed by binging is one of the characteristic traits of bulimia. Bulimia is a psychiatric disorder that involves a distinct pattern and frequency of binges (and usually purging). But binging, particularly followed by purging, does indicate a dangerous preoccupation with food, whether defined as bulimia or not.

Purging is the act of getting rid of food (or weight), and it may involve the use of diuretics (to lose water), laxatives, or vomiting. It's impossible to know just how widespread purging is in our society because people who do it often keep it a secret. But when you consider the problems involved with dieting, it's not at all surprising that purging occurs. Purging can seem like the only solution to an otherwise impossible problem—how to keep the pounds off and still eat what you want. But the fact is that even purging doesn't work! Regardless of how food is excreted, it is still absorbed; it's mostly water that's lost. And the risks involved in purging are very dangerous. Electrolyte imbalances (which can cause death), and nutritional and vitamin deficiencies all arise from purging.

Who says that dieting can't hurt? That's clearly one of the most dangerous myths around.

MYTH: I SHOULD WEIGH WHAT THE IDEAL WEIGHT TABLES TELL ME I SHOULD WEIGH

There are some serious problems involved in studying the relationship between body weight and life expectancy. And obesity researchers have been questioning the techniques used in arriving at these "ideal weights."

We all know the ideal weight tables well. They tell you the ideal weight range for someone of your particular height and frame size for maximum life expectancy. And logically enough, they were developed by the Metropolitan Life Insurance Company (see page 120). They certainly sound like something we should take pretty seriously.

But there are some important statistical problems regarding the construction of these tables that need to be examined. The tables of ideal body weight are based on accumulated data, which has been examined and interpreted, as other scientific research. The hypothesis, simply stated, is this: People who are at their ideal weight live longer than people who are not. Now, what experiments were done to prove whether or not the hypothesis is true? Well, in the case of the tables of ideal body weights, experiments have not been carried out in a laboratory with test tubes and computers. In this case, the laboratory has been the real world. And this is the problem.

In an ideal scientific experiment, everything is carefully controlled in the laboratory. Then, one item is varied and the outcome of that variation is studied. Here's an example. Say we're testing the effect that the tastiness of food has on eating behavior. We could start with two genetically identical mice and put them in the same environment. We could feed one mouse standard laboratory food, while we give the other mouse the same food but with a bitter-tasting chemical added to it. After a couple of weeks, we could weigh the two mice, and based on their weights we could make a statement about the influence of the tastiness of food on the body weight of this particular type of mouse. Then, other researchers would repeat the experiment and test the validity of the results. And if the same results came up again and again, this would be scientific knowledge that could then fit into a larger puzzle about the tastiness of food and how it affects eating behavior and body weight in a more general way. Everything in this experiment was carefully controlled except for the single variable of the bitter-tasting chemical. This is good science.

Now, let's turn back to the body weight tables. In the laboratory of the real world, we can't control variables. People aren't the same and their environments aren't the same. In fact, there are so many genetic and environmental differences that it's impossible to list or compare them. In this kind of experiment, the only thing to do is to choose a few variables and follow them in a very large sampling of people. The basic idea here is that if we use enough different people from different backgrounds and environments, the sheer force of numbers and variety will eventually even out the differences between them. And we will then be able to study the variable or variables in question, seeing any trends that result in terms of the society as a whole.

In the case of the ideal weight tables, there are problems with both the sample of people studied and the variables. The sample selection is not a selection of the society as a whole, but only of people who buy life insurance. This tilts the sample considerably. Economic, cultural, ethnic, race, religion, and sex are all variables that immediately come into the picture when talking about who buys life insurance and who doesn't.

Now, let's look at the variables that are being examined—body weight and mortality (length of life). We already know that there is a problem with body weight. The number registered on the scale does not distinguish body fat from the other weight components; this requires other types of measurements. And these other types of measurements were not used in forming the ideal weight tables. So we do not know how these tables would look if we were using the percentage of body fat, rather than total body weight, as a variable.

In addition, there's the issue of all the variables that have not been considered in this study. What if something totally different from body weight is causing overweight people to die at a particular age? Who knows? One hypothesis could be: "Repeated dieting leads to earlier death." Since we live in a society that can't tolerate obesity, it's likely that a greater percentage of overweight people will have dieted more than average-weight people. You can see the point here. Something entirely different from what is being examined could be going on, but we're not seeing it because we're not looking for it. This is exactly the sort of thing that happens when you're studying a complex topic in an uncontrolled environment.

So, how much can we trust these tables? What's now emerging from obesity studies is that it's more likely the extremes of weight—either very obese or very underweight—that causes early death.

And what is an ideal weight? In this case it's a number based on a flawed scientific experiment that many experts are questioning. These tables may still be useful as guidelines to help you compare yourself to a more or less average range of weights, and they may help you to set some weight control goals for yourself. But certainly they're far from an ideal.

MYTH: IT'S OK FOR CHILDREN AND
TEENS TO DIET

This is a particularly tragic myth. Studies have shown that even kindergarten children hold negative attitudes toward obesity. The relationship between body weight and self-esteem gets its start at a very early age. How concerned should we be about the weight of our children and teens? We should be concerned but with common sense. For the vast majority of children and teenagers, dieting is inappropriate. Weight control should be addressed through a family program of fitness and health.

Let's look at the exception first: what childhood and adolescent obesity really is. It's not known for certain whether childhood obesity always leads to adult obesity, but it's clear that obese teenagers usually become obese adults. And just as there are health risks for obese adults, there are similar risks for obese children and adolescents. The significantly overweight child must be treated by professionals who specialize in this area. Briefly, you should know that any good treatment program will involve family work and changes in behavior patterns (no more eating in front of the TV!), rather than strong attention to calorie control. Nutrition is crucial in treatment of the obese child since we are dealing with bodies that are still developing. Fortunately, obese children are in the minority (well under 10 percent of American children and teens will require treatment), but parents must be concerned. Studies now show that *more than 80 percent* of American teenage girls try to "diet." Adult behavior can be the cause. Adults today are passing their obsession with weight down to an entire generation of children and teenagers. When we weigh ourselves and respond angrily to what we see, our children hear us. At the dinner table, when new diets begin, the tension is felt by all. The hidden messages we give our children about our bodies is deeply felt. Many anorexics say that their illness began with casual remarks made by their parents (usually the father) suggesting that the daughter had better lose some weight. We tend to forget just how seriously children and teens can interpret our words and behavior. Adolescents are extremely sensitive about issues of self-worth, values, and self-esteem; and communications about body weight and self-worth can be felt deeply.

It's not at all surprising that dieting seems like a solution to the child or teen faced with the turmoil of growing up. Many teens whose genetic makeup does not naturally result in a low percentage of body fat, find themselves faced with the dilemma posed by mixed messages. The result, too often, is that these children and teens control their hunger and eating by dieting.

This is dangerous, and the average child should

never diet. The damage done can be emotional as well as physical. Children should be allowed to respond freely to hunger and fullness cues. And this includes hunger for all foods. The concept of "forbidden foods" should not be part of a child's world. This only adds to the conflicts that are part of their lives. If children are deprived of cookies and candy bars that they see their friend eating, they can quickly learn about "cheating" and "sneaking" food. It's surprising how naturally children seem to eat reasonable portions of all of the food groups when left on their own. Overconsumption of calorically rich foods usually becomes a problem because of lack of exercise, so try to direct your child's interest toward other, more physical activities.

By the time your child becomes a teenager, sensible parenting will not always work. Peer influence is so strong in a teenager's life that parents will often have a difficult time making an impact even if they try. Here you can only act in the best way possible. And there are some guidelines you can follow. The model of behavior that you set for your family is extremely important. Families that share an interest in physical activity and sports are already ahead of the game. But don't expect your teenager not to care about dieting, if you're trying every new fad diet that comes along.

Most eating disorders begin in the early teens, so *be careful*. And *be concerned*. If your teenager suddenly begins to lose a lot of weight, don't be pleased; show concern. Monitor what they're eating. Watch out for trips to the bathroom right after eating; this is when purging goes on. Also, be aware of the fact that no one is immune to drug addiction—teens included. Cocaine is a powerful appetite suppressant. Weight loss, when seen together with other behavior changes, such as change in friends, drop in grades, poor hygiene, or mood swings, could be evidence of cocaine or other drug use. So be alert.

Even healthy, "normal" kids are paying for our culture's obsession with weight and are developing a distorted sense of self-worth. Help your kids to build a good sense of self-worth. Encourage them to enjoy sports, music, clubs, and friends. If you're not focusing on the importance of self-worth, self-esteem, and positive life-style, then they probably won't either.

------------- CHAPTER -------------

4

Social and
Psychological Myths

**MYTH: IT'S NORMAL TO BE OBSESSED
WITH YOUR WEIGHT**

Can you be "normal" and "obsessed" at the same time? Doesn't obsession imply abnormality? Logic would support that view. Unfortunately, it's more usual than not for people to be obsessed with weight. So common, in fact, that it prevails in much of our society.

One problem is that "normal" is a relative term, depending on which culture is defining what the norm is. Which of these two statements is more normal to you:

#1: "I'm through dieting, I've lost enough weight."

#2: "I need to lose about five more pounds."

Certainly you've heard the second statement made more than you've heard the first. If a friend greeted you with Statement #1, you'd probably respond with surprise. This simply isn't the "normal" approach to dieting or to weight, or even to life. Statement #2, on the other hand, is much more acceptable. There's absolutely nothing surprising or abnormal about wanting to lose five more pounds (unless perhaps the statement is made by an anorexic). Remember, "You can't be too rich or too thin." That's what our society tells us. And our society also stresses achievement so strongly that we're always pushing ourselves to our limits. So, what's five more pounds? Of course that sounds normal. Feeling "finished" with any project, especially when it's a diet, is just not "normal" in our culture.

Is it normal to be a "body checker"? This does not mean checking out other people's bodies (that's an obsession in its own right); what we're referring to is checking out your own. How many times have you seen someone looking in the mirror, dissecting their bodies with their eyes? Most people do it. Perhaps you do too. Is the tummy bulging, or is it nice and flat? Have the hips gotten any smaller after exercise? How do they look from this angle or from that? You don't even really need a mirror; the hands will do (especially for the every-five-minute status reports on the stomach). This behavior is common, acceptable, and appropriate in our culture. Right?

But does it make sense? Well, that's another matter. The tummy doesn't change every five minutes. And how can fat thighs and flabby arms visibly respond to thirty minutes of aerobics?

There's something wrong with this "norm" that has so thoroughly taken over our society. That's not to say that there's no good in it. Obviously eating healthily has its benefits. But there's quality of life to consider. And we can't have it if we leave no room for a middle ground. An occasional cheeseburger and a milkshake may not be all that healthy on a daily basis (too much fat, and for some people, too many calories), but it should also not be the subject of intense internal debate. And why should the mirror be the enemy to so many and the friend to so few?

Many groups in our society have a vested interest in promoting diet obsession, but their interests are not yours and they are not medically or scientifically sound. But chic Madison Avenue styles, the television industry, the media, and the fashion designers are a lot to overcome. Can it be done? Are these cultural norms too much a part of all levels or our society? Studies show that children aged 5 to 6 view excess weight as ugly and undesirable. And when asked their opinions about overweight people children use words like "lazy," "stupid," "ugly," and "clumsy."

So, as we can see, it does seem normal to be obsessed with weight, a so-called cultural reality. But if you can practice the sound medical and nutritional principles in this book, it's possible for you not to be a victim of weight obsession. It's possible to view cultural obsession as something for someone else, and to be comfortable with yourself at the same time.

MYTH: ALL PEOPLE CAN HAVE
BEAUTIFUL BODIES IF THEY
JUST WORK AT IT

Don't you wish this were the one myth that was true? The fitness ads on TV and in magazines swear that it's possible for anyone to have a beautiful body. All it seems to take is a well-equipped gym or expensive club to transform any body into that firm, sleek, muscular look so fiercely desired today. The young men and women seen grunting, straining, and sweating to sculpt those undeniably perfect bodies could be you! Yes, the implication is that anyone can have a beautiful body, and if they don't, then they're just not working hard enough. But can six months or a year of solid exercise really make you look that good? Often the answer is no. It's another variation on the "Diet Guru" scam.

To give this some perspective, remember what it was like back when you were fourteen or fifteen years old and you were spending a day at the beach or by the pool? Your friends came in all shapes and sizes. Some people had "washboard" tummies, and some didn't. Some had long bodies with short legs, and others had just the opposite. Some legs were like tree stumps, while others tapered down to thin ankles. One thing's for sure, it wasn't aerobics or Nautilus that made those bodies different. Normal genetic variation, with perhaps some minor life-style influences, caused the variation in everyone's shape. We weren't meant to be the same. Different people have different bone structures, hip shapes, and different amounts of fat naturally placed on their buttocks and thighs. The shape of your body parts is something you're born with. To change this natural design may be difficult or even impossible.

As you've seen in earlier chapters, some parts of the body such as muscle and subcutaneous fat (fat just below the skin) will respond to exercise. But the ease and ability of making these changes is also biologically determined. And for many, the look of "today's" body is going to require tremendous amounts of time and effort (and money). The scenario often includes an intense early effort, followed by significant tapering off, discouragement and loss of interest, and general disappointment with the results. This is a tragedy. The main point of exercise should not be to make you look a certain way, but to make you feel good and healthy enough to lose weight. If you introduce a sensible physical program into your life's routine, you can greatly improve your sense of physical well-being.

What about surgery? This is certainly the latest fad. Once only facelifts, tummy tucks, and breast surgery were available. Now we have the possibility of liposuction (surgical removal of fat deposits), which has created a great stir. This frequently requested procedure is even more popular than "the nose job." But beware! This is major surgery, and the results can be disastrous. It's also quite expensive and does not promise lasting results—new fat can grow back. It works best with localized fat, and is not a quick weight loss solution for general obesity. All in all, if you really want to consider liposuction, make sure you research it thoroughly first, and be certain that you get more than one opinion before you proceed. And also, don't forget to ask yourself, *why?*

You have a body that you were born with. It's yours. Don't let the hard sell of the media determine how you mold it. Work with what God gave you and you can enjoy the rewards of sensible physical activity as part of your everyday life. You won't end up as a "model," but you will feel better if you try to become the "best you."

MYTH: FAT PEOPLE AND THIN PEOPLE ARE DIFFERENT

Researchers have found that there *are* two fundamentally different groups of people when it comes to eating behavior. The difference between these two groups, however, has nothing to do with their weights, but rather concerns their relationship to food.

Early behavioral theories about obesity proposed that fat people acted differently from thin people. Experts in behavior thought that if they taught fat people to act like thin people, their weight problems would be solved. But one by one, each of these early theories has been disproved by careful observation, testing, and experimentation. Certain behavior patterns studied, such as response to external food rather than to internal hunger cues, were found to exist not just in fat people, but in all weight classes. No predictions could be made about how overweight people would act, and the behaviorist psychologists were not successful at figuring out how to treat or train overweight people in any special way.

These types of experiments, however, were not complete failures. There have been some unexpected results that are extremely important and useful.

What we now know is that there are two types of eaters—the *restrained eater* and the *unrestrained eater*. And it is the restrained eater who has the eating problems. A restrained eater is someone who sometimes, or in more cases, always restricts the amount of food he or she eats in order to control body weight. In essence, they are chronic dieters, and they come from all weight classes.

The restrained eater is in a constant mental struggle with food. This type of eater doesn't eat when hungry and stop when satisfied. But rather, eating is a continual mental processing of the caloric volume of food ("calorie counting"). All food is either "good" or "bad." And either you are good and stick to a diet, or you're "bad" and have blown it. Once the diet is blown, restraint is abandoned and intense eating begins. This pattern explains the typical American who has a preoccupation with weight, which causes a number of serious problems.

As we've already discussed, restrictive dieting followed by binging is a method of weight control that, ironically, usually results in long-term weight gain and increase of body fat. This eating pattern leads to nutritional and emotional problems, particularly when fad diets are involved, which is often the case with the restrained eater.

Dieting is by nature extremely stressful. It involves continually fighting biological urges, coupled with guilt-ridden indulgences when hunger and deprivation can no longer be fought. This does not leave the restrained eater with a moment's peace. The result is chronic stress. The typical restrained eater is often "hyper-emotional" and suffers from anxiety and depressive symptoms, a high price to pay for weight control!

Identifying the behavior patterns of the *restrained* eater is a very important scientific breakthrough, because the physical and emotional suffering involved will end if *unrestrained* eating habits can be learned.

The *unrestrained* eater has a totally different

relationship to food. The unrestrained eater responds to internal physical signals of hunger and fullness as a guide to eating. Unrestrained eaters can be thin, average weight, or fat. Their most important trait is that weight is not an issue for them. Characteristically, they are less stressed by food, eat what they like without overindulging, and are in touch with their bodies' nutritional needs. Anyone who wants to control their weight over the long term, and be healthy and satisfied at the same time, must be an unrestrained eater.

So, fat people are not *different* from thin people. But restrained eaters *are* different from unrestrained eaters. And because most people preoccupied with weight are restrained eaters, they have to learn unrestrained eating behavior to lead more peaceful fulfilling lives.

How do you overcome restrained eating? It is possible to do. The most important step here is to get back in touch with your body. We'll explore this more in chapter 6. Your body will tell you when to eat, if you just let it.

**MYTH: OBESE PEOPLE ARE
COMPULSIVE EATERS WHO LACK
THE WILLPOWER TO RESIST
TEMPTING FOODS**

There are certain people whose chemical makeup drives them to eat more food, particularly carbohydrates. This is *not* something that is determined by willpower, but by body chemistry.

Let's face it, we think people are fat because they eat too much. We know that a thin person can eat the same amount of food or more than a fat person and stay thin because of higher Energy Expenditure. But are overweight people weak, compulsive eaters, who don't have the strength of will to resist fattening foods?

To take a look at what obesity researchers are now finding, we need to understand how the brain functions. The brain is composed of trillions of nerve cells; and the nerve cells are organized into specific groups located in specific areas. Each group controls a specific function of the body. The nerve cells do their work by sending signals to one another. Nerve cells don't touch; they're each separated by a very thin space called a synapse. The way the nerve cells send their signals is by releasing particular chemicals across the synapse. And it's the chemicals that carry these messages that are of interest to us.

There is one area, deep in the brain, that is known to control hunger and satiety (the sense of fullness and satisfaction after a meal). One of the chemicals involved in sending these particular messages is called serotonin. Serotonin is made from another chemical called tryptophan, which is an amino acid that is found in the food we eat.

Now, back to the compulsive eater. In obesity research, scientists are now finding that there is a distinct relationship between the amount of serotonin in the brain and the amount of high-carbohydrate snacks consumed. Scientists are also discovering that some people may actually have a genetic makeup that demands that they have a higher level of serotonin. And how can these people get that serotonin? From foods that raise the level of tryptophan in the brain, foods that just happen to come in the form of high-carbohydrate snacks. So it's not simply that carbohydrate cravers have no willpower, but rather that their body chemistry is asking for high-carbohydrate, calorically rich foods. This is at least one reason why some people seem to be compulsive eaters.

There's another surprising thing about serotonin. In a newly identified syndrome in psychiatry known as seasonal affective disorder (SAD), researchers are finding that there are specific psychological and physical symptoms associated with a lack of sunlight. These symptoms typically include low mood, low energy, excessive sleep, and excessive eating (frequently of carbohydrate-rich foods). Now, guess which brain chemical is involved with the body's mood regulation? Serotonin. To elevate mood, the brain elevates the serotonin level. Therefore, we can surmise that some of the compulsive eating often thought to be linked to depression for emotional reasons may actually be chemically caused.

This is all very new, and certainly carbohydrate cravers are only one subgroup of compulsive eat-

ers. There are many people who clearly overeat
out of habit, boredom, frustration, loneliness, or
just because it's fun. But let's be careful about the
myth that all obese people are compulsive eaters
who lack willpower. All obese people are not compulsive eaters. And there is a distinct subgroup of
people who eat a lot of carbohydrates because
they're responding to a true physiological need.

MYTH: FAT PEOPLE ARE EMOTIONALLY UNSTABLE

One of the most frequently cited causes for obesity is emotional instability. Believing this myth
can be a self-fulfilling prophecy. Boredom, loneliness, and frustration have all been reported as
reasons for overeating. The idea that people are
overweight because they're emotionally unstable
is simply another false assertion made about
obese people. When examined scientifically, these
psychological interpretations are found to be false.

Obese people were found to be no more emotionally unstable than any of the other weight classes.
All had their share of emotional problems.

But in the course of these studies, another pattern did emerge. This had to do with problems
that resulted from living in a society that values,
promotes, and even worships thinness. It was
found that because our society exerts so much
pressure on people to be thin, there are many peo-

ple who are forever dieting; and this, particularly when paired with a condition of low self-esteem, often develops into a mental state known as "diet mentality."

Diet mentality is not a sickness, but a best-you-can-do kind of response to the message our culture constantly gives us about being thin. It's a very difficult state of mind because it leaves us in a constant state of conflict, depression, anxiety, or guilt. Depression, because of the effects of deprivation and denial that your diet has on you. Anxiety because even when you're losing weight, you're worried about gaining it back. Or guilt, because when you do eat and gain the weight back, you think you've done something wrong and your self-worth plunges down again.

The "diet mentality" is a damaging mental state. And it may be surprising to know that not all obese people have it, and many of the people who do have it are not obese at all. Many obese people are in fact quite content with themselves, while others of varying weights can be deeply affected by cultural messages about weight control.

So, fat people are not emotionally unstable. *People that are dieting are frequently emotionally unstable*. The key here, as we've been seeing all along, is to achieve a life-style that allows you to both eat and control your weight in a stable and rational way. That, as we now know, is what it is to get smart about weight control.

MYTH: WHEN I'M THINNER, I'LL BE HAPPIER

Of all the myths, this is probably the most difficult to prove wrong. Many people truly believe this and similar myths like:

- When I'm thinner, I feel better, lighter on my feet, healthier.
- When I'm thinner, my clothes fit better, and they feel more comfortable.
- When I'm thinner, I feel attractive and sexier.

We'll start with "being lighter on your feet makes you feel better." The reality of this argument rests largely on your own starting point. If you're talking about a significantly overweight and inactive person, yes, weight loss will improve endurance. That flight of stairs will be easier and so will a run down the block. But as we've already mentioned, this has more to do with the amount of the load you're carrying around than anything else. For others it's really another story. As we've already seen, being thin does not necessarily imply being fit. Even though the flight of stairs will become easier if you become lighter on your feet, this does not mean that you are fit. Health-promoting fitness comes from cardiovascular conditioning (through aerobic exercise) and muscle coordination.

Weight loss, if not conducted carefully and sensibly, can in fact lead to fatigue and malnutrition.

What about clothes fitting better and feeling more comfortable. This idea comes more from the choice of clothing you wear than it does from any kind of connection between your weight and your clothes. The simple truth is that anyone can feel comfortable in their clothes if they're willing to buy the right size. It's not unusual for people to buy clothes that are too tight in the hope of fitting into them later. Another common mistake comes in buying clothes at the end of a successful diet, only to find that it's impossible to keep the weight off and to stay in the clothes comfortably. The clothes then turn into a symbol of failure.

Let's examine the third statement, "when I'm thinner, I feel attractive and sexier." This is a tough one to debunk because, again, it relates to society's standard of what these qualities mean. Television and magazines tell us that thin is sexy and attractive. Unfortunately, this tends to make the weight-conscious person feel less sexy and attractive while they're trying to lose weight. And attractiveness and sexiness is, at least in part, a state of mind. You have assets of your own, and buying into society's notion of things only devalues what you have. A low estimation of your own value is communicated to others in many different ways; others pick up on your negativity and get turned off, and the situation gets worse. Your internal belief that you're not sexy or attractive is confirmed *not* because of what others believe, but because of what you believe.

Physical attractiveness and sexiness largely depend on promoting what you've got. Did you ever see a famous model or movie star without their makeup and fancy clothes? The right clothes and makeup can do wonders for you no matter what your weight is. If you're waiting to get thin to be glamorous, then it's no wonder you cling to the belief that thin people are sexy and attractive.

All these myths about thinness and happiness are largely based on self-defeating behaviors and attitudes you may form when you're not thin. And even if you do lose all the weight you think you must lose, your *body image* still may not improve. Body image is your own personal perception of your body. A common problem is to see yourself as being larger than you really are. This distorted view often leads to an intense desire to lose weight that may be out of proportion with reality. Just think of all the people you know who call themselves "fat" when they don't look fat at all. It is their own internal body image that tells them they are fat, not reality.

Pinning your happiness to weight loss is a risky matter. Acquisition of material or physical objects rarely leads to true happiness. Happiness does, however, come in the form of peace of mind. Release yourself from the grip of body weight obsession, and peace of mind can be your reward. Again, get smart. Strive for a comfortable life-style with achievable levels of calorie control and exercise. That will make you happier—you'll be making the best of what you've got.

----------- CHAPTER -------------

5

Today's "Hot" Myths and Fads

MYTH: SUGAR IS BAD FOR YOU

Do you believe that if you stop eating sweets, you'll lose twenty pounds? Most people do. In fact, sugar is the number-one ingredient on people's "forbidden foods" list. Many believe that sugar is the direct cause of weight gain. It's also been blamed for hyperactivity in children and hypoglycemia in adults. Add to that, the "tooth decay factor," and you're left with a deadly enemy indeed. But, in fact, sugar is not the villain that people imagine.

Chemically speaking, sugars are carbohydrates that happen to taste sweet. There are various types of sugar. Glucose and fructose molecules combine to form sucrose, the most common sugar. Fruit sugar is strictly fructose. Sugar is found in many forms and products such as honey and molasses. And all of them share a common property— they have no nutritional value. This means that they do nothing to contribute chemically or struc-

turally to the body's functioning (except to contribute fuel to run other processes). Sugar is
essentially a neutral substance. It is neither toxic
nor disease-promoting. So why all the fuss?

Let's start with an old favorite—tooth decay. Although sugar feeds the bacteria that cause tooth
decay, it doesn't mean that the only way to fight
tooth decay is to cut out sugar. All you have to do
is brush and floss, because by itself, sugar does not
cause tooth decay.

Another popular misconception about sugar is
that it causes hyperactivity in children. Parents,
overwhelmed with the difficulties of child-rearing,
are eager to grasp at something that might reduce
(or at least explain) the intense activity characteristic of growing children. Once it was suggested
that excess sugar might be the cause of hyperactivity, it became a self-fulfilling prophecy. They
believed that increased sugar directly caused hyperactivity in their children, and then "observed"
it to be true. Since this sort of prejudiced observation has long been a problem in scientific experimentation, scientists have developed what is
known as "double blind" study. When double blind
experiments were conducted in hyperactive children, there was absolutely *no association* seen between sugar intake and energy level.

Similarly, people would love to believe that
moodiness and anxiety is linked to sugar intake;
this could explain many "fad" diseases, such as
hypoglycemia. Hypoglycemia occurs when an in-

take of concentrated sugar causes a rapid rise in plasma insulin, which then leads to the rapid removal of sugar from the bloodstream, resulting in shakiness, moodiness, anxiety, and inability to concentrate. A few years ago, millions of people were being diagnosed as hypoglycemic, all being put on special diets to "balance out" blood sugar.

Hypoglycemia is a physiological condition, and the treatment prescribed *does* make some sense. But this condition is *very rare,* and has been overdiagnosed. The only way it can be diagnosed accurately is to measure blood sugar at the time the person has hypoglycemic symptoms. Low blood sugar without symptoms is simply a variation on normal and means very little.

Are sugar and weight control connected? Certainly there is cause for concern, but not necessarily for the reasons you may have thought. Sugar by itself is not where the bulk of the calories consumed lies.

Human beings (and other animals) like a sweet taste; the tongue has its own special receptors that immediately detect sweetness and send it right to the brain. Food producers, not surprisingly, have seized on this fact, and to satisfy consumers, they place a good deal of sugar in most foods. The thing that makes sweets potentially dangerous is not necessarily the sugar, but the fact that they are calorically rich. The rule of thumb is: Where there is sugar in sweets there is also usually fat.

So, the foods to stay away from if you're thinking about calorie intake are not necessarily those that have sugar, but those that have fat. This is not to say that they are "forbidden foods." If you want to satisfy your natural desire for sweetness, fruit can often meet the need. A slice of cake or a candy bar is okay, too, but from time to time, as long as you're getting most of your calories from sensible meals.

MYTH: HIGH-PROTEIN, LOW-CARBOHYDRATE DIETS PROMOTE RAPID, PERMANENT WEIGHT LOSS

Despite the fact that it isn't true, this myth has been around for a long time, and doesn't seem to fade. First seen in the book *Calories Don't Count,* published in 1960, it has since appeared in varying forms. *Dr. Atkin's Diet Revolution, The Doctor's Quick Weight Loss Diet,* and *The Complete Scarsdale Medical Diet,* among others. The popularity of these approaches to dieting is based on a number of commonly observed patterns and misconceptions promoted by their proponents. Some of these are:

1. *Quick results.* Low-carbohydrate diets, as we've already discussed, result in rapid initial weight loss. By removing carbohydrates from the diet, you overload the bloodstream with protein and fat, creating an imbalance. This imbalance then produces toxins, and to fight the toxins, the body shifts a large amount of water from the cells into the bloodstream to flush them out. The result of this is water loss through urination, which is seen as rapid weight loss. This is more attractive than the slow loss of fat because of low calorie intake, which is not all that noticeable compared to the five to ten pounds of water lost during the first week of a typical low-carbohydrate diet.

2. *The "magic" of protein.* The myth that it takes extra calories to digest protein has been disproved many times, but for some reason it refuses to die. It was once believed that nearly all the protein calories consumed were burned up in the digestion process, making protein almost a "free food." This was referred to as the "specific dynamic action" of protein. If this were true it would be a great way to lose weight. But it's not. Protein offers no special advantage over fats and carbohydrates in terms of the amount of calories used in digestion.

3. *Protein is good for you.* This myth derives from the fact that lean body tissue, including muscle, is mostly made of protein. But it is a faulty assumption that eating protein builds muscles. The truth is that it's necessary to eat protein to supply the body with certain required amino acids, which are important for many body processes,

muscle-building among them. But muscle-building itself happens only when the muscles are exercised, and the energy required to do this can come not only from protein but from any kind of food.

4. *Low-carbohydrate diets result in ketosis, a state in which fat is rapidly burned off.* When the body does not receive enough carbohydrates, it's also not getting the glucose it needs as fuel. So to compensate, it turns to burning fat almost exclusively. This produces toxic chemicals called ketones. And when ketones are being produced, the body is in the "state of ketosis." There's a common belief that ketosis is desirable because it leads to increased energy and decreased appetite. Scientific studies, however, have generally proved this to be untrue. Ketosis, while it may help in short-term weight loss, is in fact an unnatural state that can lead to significant medical complications. And while the energy burned in ketosis is almost exclusively from fat, this does *not* mean that your excess body fat is necessarily being tapped—it's burned calories that count. So there are no particular advantages to putting your body in this unnatural condition. You're only depriving yourself of the balanced nutrition your body needs and wants.

5. *The protein-sparing modified fast.* Fasting is a dangerous, albeit rapid, way to lose weight. With no food coming in, the body receives no glucose and is forced to rely in part on muscle tissue to make it run. It's also not getting the necessary amino acids, and it must rely on the muscles for this too. During fasting, as much as 50 percent of the weight lost is from muscle tissue (and some tissue from body organs).

At one time, physicians interested in weight loss speculated that if the body could get some amino acids from eating just a small amount of protein, many of the negative effects of fasting could be reversed. This theory resulted in the "protein-sparing" diet (body protein is spared by eating some pure protein daily). This was originally intended for the morbidly obese (more than 100 pounds over the ideal body weight) and involved very low daily caloric intake (about 300 to 400). As is often the case, this specialized diet was quickly commercialized, becoming the now notorious Last Chance Diet. Liquid and powdered protein diets based on the protein-sparing principle are still popular today.

There's no denying that you lose weight from these diets, but you also risk serious nutritional and mineral deficiencies, and electrolyte imbalances. And even when you manage to avoid medical complications, these extremely low-calorie diets usually result in weight gain in the long run. Once the diet has ended, you're left with a very low basal metabolic rate, and usually the eating that follows is not normal. A diet that involves this degree of deprivation is the classic setup for binging. Nonetheless, as we have seen, the protein-sparing diet initially looks like it does the trick, continuing to lend mystique to the importance of protein in weight loss. So, be smart, and be careful, and avoid this type of diet.

Protein's role in diet history has been long and varied. And with so many sources, the myth that protein has some special and even magical qualities when it comes to weight loss will probably live on for a long time. Protein is no more than a type of food required by the body—there's nothing magic about it. The body needs protein, just as it needs carbohydrates and fat for sensible, long-term weight control.

**MYTH: CELLULITE IS A SPECIAL KIND
        OF FAT REQUIRING SPECIAL
        TREATMENT**

Cellulite is a different kind of body fat, but it requires no special treatment. In that sense, it is the same as any other fat. Again, the myth makers are looking for your dollars.

Cellulite—those puckered, orange-peel-like deposits of fat we all dread—is most frequently seen on women's thighs and buttocks. America's quest for "smooth," "tight," and "firm" makes us particularly attentive to ridding ourselves of cellulite, to the point that there is now an entire industry devoted to its removal. We take ourselves to glamorous, often European-style spas and are bathed, wrapped, massaged, electrified, and injected, hopefully emerging with thin thighs and tight backsides! But here again, it's not possible.

When it comes to cellulite, there are two major forces involved. One has to do with the orange-peel look, and the other with the tendency for this particular fat to be pocketed in women's thighs and buttocks. First, we'll examine the orange-peel look.

The thing that makes cellulite different, and that gives it its characteristic appearance, is not the fat itself but the connective tissue surrounding the fat. Connective tissue is a substance that binds things together and holds them in their place. We're all familiar with elastic tissue—the tissue that holds the skin tight and that cause wrinkles when it loosens. People who have lost a lot of weight know what happens when this tissue loses some of its elasticity, at least initially after weight loss. As we age, elastic tissue weakens and wrinkles appear. And, despite all claims to the contrary, there is little we can do to reverse or slow down this process. There is no magical, or even sensible, way to affect connective tissue. And this includes the connective tissue that is part of cellulite.

The other factor at work in the case of cellulite involves evolution. Over millions of years, women have adaptively evolved fat deposits that could be saved and depended upon during times of need, when extra fuel might be required. And most women hold these deposits in their thighs and buttocks. This is something that is genetically determined.

There is a way to reduce these fat deposits, but to do this, it's necessary to reduce the body fat in total. Unfortunately, the thighs and buttocks seem to be the most difficult areas to reduce. These fat cells have different membrane properties that make the body reluctant to give them up. We have all seen the results of a dieter fighting her body's natural inclination to store this fat— the body that is skinny on top (sometimes to the point of appearing like a skeleton), while the lower body firmly holds on to its noticeable fat deposits.

The puckered look is part of the connective tissue attached to it, something that can't be changed. And as far as getting rid of cellulite from the thighs and buttocks, that's just where extra fat tends to reside in women, something genetically determined as a result of millions of years of evolution. More often than not, the fat you'd most like to lose is the last to go. So, if you want cellulite to go, it has to be part of your own overall weight loss program, not a goal in itself.

MYTH: IT'S POSSIBLE TO BE ADDICTED
TO FOOD

You cannot be "hooked" on food, or on a particular food, in the same way that a drug addict is
"hooked" on drugs. While it may feel like certain
foods are impossible to resist and make you break
any weight control program you try, there is no
such thing as a "food addiction."

The major confusion regarding so-called food
addiction comes from scientific research now being conducted on a syndrome known as "eater's
high." To understand "eater's high" (not unlike
"runner's high"), you have to know something
about the body's endogenous, or naturally occur-
ing, opiates.

Heroin, codeine, morphine, and other similarly
dangerous drugs all belong to a class of chemicals
known as opiates. They have a powerful effect on
the brain, causing intense pleasure and euphoria
(and addiction.) When researchers began to look
into why these drugs have the effect they do, they
discovered that there are cells in the brain that
are specifically designed to respond to opiates
known as receptors. This enabled scientists to find
endogenous opiates, similar chemicals that occur
naturally in the brain. This discovery has helped
us to understand the body's internal pleasure and
reward system; why we "feel" good when we eat,

make love, participate in sports, even get a pat on the shoulder from the boss.

One specific internal reward comes from eating. Experts theorize that obese people's eating behaviors cause an exaggerated endogenous opiate response, referred to as "eater's high." Consequently, scientists decided that if you blocked the endogenous opiate effect, obese people might lose weight. Experiments were conducted with a drug that blocks endogenous opiates, but weight did not change. Obese people were simply *not* physically addicted to food.

There is, however, more research going on in this field, and this may have some significance in treating bulimia. At Fair Oaks Hospital, and elsewhere, doctors experimenting with "eater's high" are finding that opiate-blocking drugs can work to decrease the intensity and frequency of binges in some bulimics. This research holds promise regarding a certain percentage of bulimics, but it does not apply to the population at large. And anyone who binges is not necessarily bulimic; bulimia is a psychiatric illness with many other specific symptoms attached to it, and a subject worthy of at least an entire book.

Trying to justify behavior as food addiction only distracts us from the real issues. The simple reason you feel excessively attached to certain foods is because they're usually the ones you deny yourself on a diet. This is not a physiological need, but a basic psychological one, clearly related to the self-defeating "forbidden food" concept. You may be mentally preoccupied with food, but that is by no means an addiction. Don't be lured into thinking it is, just to justify poor eating habits.

MYTH: IDENTIFYING FOOD ALLERGIES CAN HELP TO CONTROL WEIGHT

There is no scientific basis for the concept of "food allergies" when it comes to weight control. "Food allergy" is another scientific-sounding term to help explain away some of our health and weight problems. Some diet doctors now offer batteries of tests to diagnose and treat allergies to nearly everything imaginable. After all, many people think if their eating, fitness, energy, and health problems can be linked to a particular food, then the cure should be easy; and if it's not, then they're not to blame, it's an allergy. If you think this all sounds too easy to be true, you're right, it is.

To understand why this concept makes no sense, let's look at how a real allergy like hay fever works. In the case of hay fever, your body mistakenly thinks that pollen is an infection and works to fight it off. But with pollen, unlike a real danger like bacteria or a virus, the body is sometimes misprogrammed and responds negatively to a substance that is in fact not harmful or invasive.

One of the ways in which the body typically

fights infections is with a special cell called the mast cell. This cell is essentially like a plastic bag filled with histamine, a chemical that aids in fighting infections. Most of the time, antibodies on the surface of the mast cell tell it when an enemy is approaching, which then leads it to release the histamine. Histamine causes symptoms such as rashes, a runny nose, nasal congestion, watery eyes, and itching—all of which you may recognize as conditions of an allergy. And when the mast cells respond mistakenly to pollen, the result is hay fever. We treat true allergies with antihistamines, decongestants, and other drugs, sometimes in the form of allergy shots over a one-to two-year period in more serious cases.

However, allergies are now being mistakenly considered as the cause of a whole new range of problems—most notably psychological and weight control related—which have no basis in science. Food is part of the list of substances that might cause such an allergic response, and certain foods can cause real allergic reactions. Allergies to shellfish, for example, are particularly common. But the symptoms of these reactions are histamine-mediated responses such as rashes, itching, breathing difficulty, nausea, vomiting, and diarrhea—not the psychological, behavioral, and weight-related conditions now being proposed by the "food allergy" fad.

"Food allergists" say that you can trace the cessation of a particular symptom, such as fatigue or irritability, to the removal of a particular food from the diet. The food must be removed completely, or neutralized by food extracts for a complex reintroduction back into the diet. The "sufferer" then experiences revived health, including weight loss and increased energy. Sounds good! But there's absolutely no science behind it.

Food, of course, is the chief culprit in this latest scheme of the "pseudo-scientists." Science has shown there are food intolerances in some people. There are definitely passing symptoms, such as bloating and gastrointestinal upset, that may be caused by specific foods. But there is no scientific evidence to indicate that these "food allergies" cause significant health problems (other than the histamine-mediated responses noted above).

If a serious physical or psychological problem such as fatigue, depression, or irritability develops, check it out. A doctor can help you find the source of your problem through scientific means, and cure you by taking the appropriate steps.

MYTH: FOOD COMBINATIONS AND SPECIAL FOOD SCHEDULES CAN LEAD TO FAT LOSS THROUGH SPECIAL PROCESSES

There's no scientific research at all suggesting that the body responds to changing the time, order, or combination in which foods are eaten. The only possible reason for this fad comes from our willingness to accept holistic or "total health" plans. The holistic outlook often seems more "humane," promising total health from life-style and dietary changes. But it's another empty magic bullet.

The most popular programs are the Beverly Hills Diet and the Fit for Life plan. Both of these regimens are complex; they demand great time and effort, and they promise magical results. They refer to special fat-burning enzymes, and special assimilation and elimination cycles in the body. Both, interestingly enough, also advise that you eat a lot of fruit and drink a lot of water. Understanding simple physiology is important before trying these diets.

Eating large amounts of fruit, or only fruit, usually causes diarrhea. Diarrhea is bowel movement with high water content, which causes the food to move quickly through the intestines. Calories, however, are not blocked from entering the body in this process. Definitely there is weight lost, but once again, it's water weight, not fat. This loss of water weight is further encouraged by extra urination caused by all the water you're supposed to be drinking.

Besides loss of water weight, these diets encourage low calorie intake based on the old monotony trick. If you can only eat from one food class, then of course you're going to get tired of it. Take a diet that lets you eat all the steak you want, but nothing more over a period of time. Now steak is a calorically rich food, but when eaten exclusively without a buttered potato, bread, and butter, and a salad surrounding it, it loses some of its appeal; chances are, you'll eat less of it than you would under other circumstances.

This monotony factor results in initial weight loss but is the reason why these diets fail over a long period of time. The dieter normally responds to the wide variety of foods available. And diets that require that we ignore this reality can only work for a small group of people.

Cross these fad diets off altogether. There's no scientific research behind them.

MYTH: FAD DIETS WORK!

Actually, fad diets do work for some people. The first few pages of any fad diet book will quote one successful dieter after another, all praising this particular diet and telling how it worked for them. And, yes, the diet did work for these people. But that's more the result of the particular people who succeeded than the result of diet. Statistical probability tells us that in a society obsessed with weight loss, there is bound to be a small percentage of the population ready to commit to *any* diet seriously. And because fad diets involve decreased caloric intake, weight will inevitably be lost by this small group.

The people who have success stories typically tell their friends, the diet's reputation spreads by word of mouth. It will be the latest fad—that is, until the enthusiasm dies. Then the next diet comes along, and the same thing happens again. And with this, one fad diet replaces another. Once the diet has spread beyond the original enthusiastic group, the new group will not necessarily be as motivated for the commitment that success entails.

Why has there never been one fad diet plan that works for a large number of people for a long period of time? It's not just because nearly all fad diets require extreme changes in eating habits that are impossible to maintain. The truth is that there's really no one diet plan waiting to be discovered, because deep down everyone knows what that plan is already. It may not be magical or catchy, but it works. *To lose weight and keep it off, long-term, lifelong eating and physical activity patterns must be changed: Cut back on calories, eat a balanced diet, and exercise. It's simple.* When you *get smart* about weight control, it's easy to see that fad diets never work! True health and happiness come from attending to all parts of your life: you can do your best at work, fully appreciate your family, and enjoy being you. And this can all come with an intelligent approach to weight control—one that takes into account your own genetic background and helps you to set realistic goals.

**MYTH: IF A WEIGHT CONTROL PRODUCT
IS ON THE MARKET, IT MUST BE
SAFE; THE FEDERAL GOVERN-
MENT REGULATES THEM**

It may surprise you to learn that many weight
control products simply do not require Food and
Drug Administration (FDA) approval. And for
those weight control products that do require FDA
approval, pharmaceuticals, for example, the possibility exists that FDA approval will not guarantee the long-term safety of the product.

Liquid protein diets are a tragic example.

In the seventies, liquid-protein preparations
were the rage. This fad diet promised rapid and
permanent weight loss. No FDA approval was
necessary because liquid protein was considered
to be a nutritional supplement not a drug. Popularity of liquid protein finally ebbed during
FDA and Centers for Disease Control investiga-
tions, but only after deaths resulted from their
use. (Although the reason for these deaths is still
not fully understood, the concept of liquid diets
is still alive; they've been improved, and are
clearly more nutritionally sound than before, although the long-term effectiveness is still open
to serious question.)

Conversely, because the FDA has granted approval does not necessarily guarantee that the

SUMMARY OF POPULAR DIETARY APPROACHES TO WEIGHT CONTROL

approach	characteristics	examples*
moderate caloric restriction	Usually 1,000–1,800 kcal per day Reasonable balance of macronutrients Encourage exercise May employ behavioral approach	The Setpoint Diet Slim Chance in a Fat World Weight Watcher's Diet The American Heart Association Diet Mary Helen's Help Yourself Diet Plan
low carbohydrate	Less than 100 gm carbohydrate per day	Atkin's Diet Revolution Calories Don't Count Drinking Man's Diet Woman Doctor's Diet for Women The Doctor's Quick Weight Loss Diet (Stillman's) The Complete Scarsdale Medical Diet
low fat	Less than 20% of calories from fat Limited (or elimination of) animal protein sources, all fats, nuts, seeds	The Rice Diet Report The Macrobiotic Diet The Pritikin Diet
novelty diets	Promote certain nutrients, foods, or combination of foods as having unique, magical, or previously undiscovered qualities	Dr. Berger's Immune Power Diet Fit for Life Diet The Rotation Diet The Beverly Hills Diet
very-low-calorie diets	Less than 800 kcal per day Also known as protein-sparing modified fasts	Optifast Cambridge Diet The Last Chance Diet The Rotation Diet Genesis
formula diets	Based on formulated or packaged products Many are very-low-calorie diet regimens (see above)	U.S.A. (United Sciences of America), Inc. Optifast Genesis Cambridge Diet Herbalife The Last Chance Diet Slimfast

*Diets may be listed in more than one category if multiple characteristics apply.

From: JOURNAL OF THE AMERICAN DIETETIC ASSOCIATION, Jan. 1988

COMPARISON OF DIETS TO DIETARY GOALS

(Percent distribution of energy sources)

■ % PROTEIN □ % FAT □ % CARBOHYDRATE

DIETS	CALORIES	% Protein	% Fat	% Carbohydrate
DIETARY GOALS			30	55
Beverly Hills	928	4		90
F-Diet	1241		20	62
Pritikin 1200	1273		9	66
Pritikin 700	737		10	60
I ♥ America	1307		29	46
Simmons	924		29	45
I ♥ New York	980		30	38
Scarsdale	1014		31	41
Atkins	2031		73	4
Stillman	1316		49	5

0%   25%   50%   75%   100%

Data compiled by Dr. Paul A. La Chance, and
Michelle C. Fisher, R.D., Rutgers University, 1983.

product will be used in a safe and effective manner. One example is amphetamines, a class of pharmaceutical drugs used in weight control for more than fifty years.

Originally intended to act as a mood elevator, amphetamines had one very interesting side effect: weight loss. As a diet product, amphetamines have been extremely popular with the physicians who prescribed them (often thoughtlessly) and the patients who eagerly consumed them. After all, not only were amphetamines considered by consumers to be safe (you got them from the doctor), but they had the additional advantage of elevating your mood and giving you increased energy. True, sometimes they could make you jittery or raise your blood pressure, and after a while, you'd begin to crave them and feel sluggish when there weren't any left. But how could they not be safe? The government had approved them.

The fact is that amphetamines are powerful and addictive drugs that have profound physiological effects on both the brain and the body. They are now *illegal* as a weight control prescription, and even in other areas of medicine, their use has become severely limited. But only during the last decade have amphetamines actually been fully regulated; for forty years these dangerous drugs circulated freely. The reasons for this are complex. The point, however, is clear. The American public was not protected from this hazardous product by either the FDA or by physicians.

Finally, and perhaps most alarmingly, there are popular weight control products with proven physiological and psychological dangers that continue to be on the market today—the FDA still allows them to be sold over the counter. Phenylpropanolamine (PPA)—a drug chemically similar to amphetamine—is a good example of this. PPA is the chief active ingredient in over-the-counter diet pills—yes, the ones with the snappy names sold in bright boxes and fancy displays at your local drugstore.

First of all, these pills don't work overtime; and second, they can be dangerous. In controlled experiments testing phenylpropanolamine's appetite suppressant qualities, any positive results have been negligible, or minor at best. And even any minor effect is generally short-lived (correlating with the short span in which the dieter is most motivated).

They are very dangerous. There have been numerous documented side effects resulting from PPA pills—symptoms similar to those associated with amphetamines, such as excess nervous stimulation, hypertension, anxiety, and even psychosis. A number of these problems have occurred in children and teenagers, who clearly have free access to these diet suppressants. While the FDA limits the amount of PPA per pill, this offers minor protection at best. After all, what's to stop consumers from taking whatever quantity of pills they think it will take to do the job? Why the FDA doesn't ban these pills, or at least make them available by prescription only, is unclear.

Consumer, beware! Common sense and extreme caution is essential when it comes to any new product that promises weight loss. You simply can't depend on outside forces to be doing this job for you. And, no matter what, stay away from appetite suppressants. As you'll understand by the time you've finished this book, using any artificial or chemical substance to change your eating habits might result in temporary weight loss, but without exception, it will defeat your quest for permanent weight control that fits comfortably with your life-style.

Designing Your Own Weight Control Program

By now you should be a lot smarter about weight control than you were. You've learned that there are no simple solutions, shortcuts, or magic. You now understand that the body is a wonderfully complex machine, designed to survive and not to easily shed pounds. With all of this knowledge, you're now ready to take some very important steps. You can develop your own long-term weight control program—a plan to suit your personal needs and life-style. All that it's going to take is four steps.

STEP ONE: STOP AND THINK

That's right, what you need to do first is to stop and consider everything you've just learned. Being smart is the key to all the other steps you'll be taking. So let's have a quick review, and to see how much information you've really absorbed, begin by answering the next twenty-nine true/false questions.

1. The basal metabolism accounts for up to 70 percent of the energy expended by the body every day.   True/False

2. Serotonin is a brain chemical that is important in determining whether the body is hungry or full and satisfied.   True/False

3. One pound of fat equals 3,500 calories.
                                                                                                           True/False

4. Protein and carbohydrates have the same amount of calories per gram.   True/False

5. It's best to weigh yourself at most once a week.   True/False

6. A Nautilus workout is a type of aerobic exercise.   True/False

7. Liposuction can be used to remove fat from all over the body.   True/False

8. Obese people are at greater risk of heart attack during exercise than thin people.
                                                                                                           True/False

9. An "obligate exerciser" is similar to an anorexic.   True/False

10. Diabetes can be improved by weight loss.
                                                                                                           True/False

11. A person's setpoint is determined only by genetic factors.   True/False

12. Genetics is less important than environment in determining adult body weight.
                                                                                                           True/False

13. Purging, while abnormal, is an effective way to control weight.   True/False

14. Being extremely underweight is statistically linked to shorter life expectancy.

                                        True/False

15. Childhood dieting has resulted in cases of stunted growth.   True/False

16. In our culture, obsession with dieting is an accepted behavior.   True/False

17. An hour a day is what it takes for anyone to build a firm, trim body.   True/False

18. "Restrained eaters" are often hyper-emotional.   True/False

19. Some compulsive eaters eat to raise the serotonin level in the brain.   True/False

20. The "diet mentality" is the only way to keep yourself from gaining weight.

                                        True/False

21. Body image distortion is rare in thin people.   True/False

22. If you're anxious and jittery sometimes, you're probably hypoglycemic.   True/False

23. It takes more energy to digest protein than it does to digest carbohydrates and fats.

                                        True/False

24. With special exercises, you can tone the connective tissue that causes cellulite.

                                        True/False

25. "Runner's high" and "eater's high" are exactly the same.   True/False

26. Some people have classic allergic responses to some foods.   True/False

27. "All you can eat of one food" type of diets rely on monotony to aid in weight loss.

True/False

28. If you keep searching and trying, you can eventually find a diet that works for you.

True/False

29. Phenylpropanolamine, the active ingredient in over-the-counter diet pills, is harmful in ways similar to amphetamines.

True/False

ANSWERS

1. True 2. True 3. True 4. True 5. True 6. False 7. False 8. False 9. True 10. True 11. False 12. False 13. False 14. True 15. True 16. True 17. False 18. True 19. True 20. False 21. False 22. False 23. False 24. False 25. False 26. True 27. True 28. False 29. True

How did you do? If your score was 25–29, you learned a lot. If you scored 20–24, it means you've missed some important points. And a score below 20 suggests that you need to go back and review some of the information. The questions are numbered to match up with the myths. So go back and reread the ones you've missed. The most important diet message we have today is that a good understanding of current scientific knowledge is crucial in designing any long-term weight control program that works.

STEP TWO: BUY CLOTHES

If you don't have a comfortable set of clothes, then go out and get one now. No more squeezing yourself into the wrong size. You can't possibly begin any sensible weight loss program if your clothes are demanding that you lose weight fast. This is going to be a long process, and you're going to need to be comfortable if you want it to work. Your first goal will be to learn what it is to feel physically at ease with your body, even before you actually begin to lose weight.

STEP THREE: EXERCISE

Yes, exercise comes next. This step is the most important one when it comes to getting yourself to break the "diet mentality" and control your weight. Start your exercise program before you begin to think about changing your eating habits. *Do not cut calories. Do not diet.* First put exercise into your daily routine. Here are some questions to ask yourself that will help you do it.

1. Do you need a medical evaluation first? It is a good idea to see your doctor before starting an exercise program, especially if you meet any of the following criteria:

a. Anyone with a history of heart or lung problems.

b. Anyone over thirty-five who has never seriously exercised before.

c. Anyone with a family history of heart disease or high blood pressure.

d. Anyone who has current problems with hypertension, diabetes, high blood cholesterol, or triglycerides, or with cigarette smoking.

e. Anyone who is more than 40 percent over ideal body weight.

2. Ask yourself, what kind of exercise is best for me? The exercise you do must be aerobic. You'll be putting together a plan in which you exercise at least four times a week for 30 minutes at a time, so you're going to have to think seriously about what you're going to be most comfortable doing. Remember, the long term is your goal. The following is a chart that lists different aerobic activities and the number of calories they burn per minute.

As you can see, there are lots of choices. Decide which are the best activities for you. And when you've chosen, pay careful attention to the following: The steps below are based on material created by Barry A. Franklin, Ph.D. ("Exercise Program Compliance," *Behavioral Management of Obesity,* edited by Storlie, JS and Jordan, HA, Spectrum Publications, Inc. Jamaica, NY 1984).

CALORIES USED PER MINUTE
DURING ACTIVITY

Activity	Weight in Pounds						
	100	120	150	170	200	220	250
Badminton	4.3	5.2	6.5	7.4	8.7	9.6	10.9
Bicycling, 5.5 mph	3.1	3.8	4.7	5.3	6.3	6.9	7.9
Bicycling, 10 mph	5.4	6.5	8.1	9.2	10.8	11.9	13.6
Calisthenics	3.3	3.9	4.9	5.6	6.6	7.2	8.2
Canoeing, 4 mph	4.6	5.6	7.0	7.9	9.3	10.2	11.6
Golf	3.6	4.3	5.4	6.1	7.2	7.9	9.0
Handball	6.3	7.6	9.5	10.7	12.7	13.9	15.8
Mountain climbing	6.6	8.0	10.0	11.3	13.3	14.6	16.6
Jogging, 11-min. mile	6.1	7.3	9.1	10.4	12.2	13.4	15.3
Running, 8-min. mile	9.4	11.3	14.1	16.0	18.8	20.7	23.5
Running, 5-min. mile	13.1	15.7	19.7	22.3	26.3	28.9	32.8
Racquetball	6.3	7.6	9.5	10.7	12.7	13.9	15.8
Skating, moderate	3.6	4.3	5.4	6.1	7.2	7.9	9.0
Skiing, downhill	6.3	7.6	9.5	10.7	12.7	13.9	15.8
Skiing, cross-country	7.2	8.7	10.8	12.3	14.5	15.9	18.0
Squash	6.8	8.1	10.2	11.5	13.6	14.9	17.0
Swimming, breaststroke	4.8	5.7	7.2	8.1	9.6	10.5	12.0
Swimming, crawl	5.8	6.9	8.7	9.8	11.6	12.7	14.5
Table tennis	2.7	3.2	4.0	4.6	5.4	5.9	6.8
Tennis	4.5	5.4	6.8	7.7	9.1	10.0	11.4
Volleyball, moderate	2.3	2.7	3.4	3.9	4.6	5.0	5.7
Walking, 3 mph	2.7	3.2	4.0	4.6	5.4	5.9	6.8
Walking, 4 mph	3.9	4.6	5.8	6.6	7.8	8.5	9.7

Developed under standardized conditions at the Human Performance Research Center at Brigham Young University in Provo, Utah.

a. *Instruction and encouragement.* There are lots of resources available to you: books, videotapes, and—probably best of all—health club instructors. They can educate, motivate, and encourage you in your exercise program.

b. *Regular routine.* At first, it's going to be difficult to get yourself to exercise regularly. But since you won't be starving yourself or constantly checking your status on the scale, it should make things a little easier. Start slowly, but not too slowly. Your instructor and other resources will help you to build up your aerobic heart rate. Find time. You may think that time is the most difficult problem. But the fact is that you can always find the time. Most people find it easiest to make time in the morning. You can always wake up a little earlier—just go to sleep a little earlier if you need to. One way to save some time is to exercise at home. This eliminates the time it takes to travel to a health or fitness club. It's all part of your "informed" decision.

c. *Freedom from injury.* Even the most motivated exerciser can be stopped by an injury. There are ways to avoid injury that you should consider. Proper clothing, shoes, and equipment are all important. Also, injuries increase with greater duration and intensity of exercise. So increase your pace slowly. Remember, you have plenty of time ahead, and moderation is always best.

d. *Enjoyment, fun, and variety.* This is very important! You won't stick to anything for long if there's no enjoyment in it. And while you'll find that aerobic exercise may be difficult at first, and that it does require regular commitment and tolerance, you'll also find that the more you're in shape, the more possibilities you'll have for variety and fun. Once you feel more secure with your physical abilities, you'll be ready for competitive games like racquetball, handball, and tennis. These sports all provide good aerobic workouts. They're not good to start with because they demand being able to keep the ball in play for a good workout. But they can be a goal to keep in mind. And when you're ready, these games can be a nice reward.

e. *Group camaraderie.* This can be key to your exercise program. A group can offer you basic support and psychological motivation in your workout. A group is also helpful in promoting regular attendance.

f. *Progress testing and recording.* Keep a record of what you're doing, and you'll be pleased to see yourself improve. Here again, a good instructor can be one of your best resources. You can chart your exercise progress in various ways. One possibility is to keep a cumulative record of all your exercise—a total of all the miles you've run, swum, bicycled, or rowed. You can also record your fitness progress by keeping track of how much faster you can do a particular activity as time passes. The many new exercise machines are another good tool for registering your improvement. These machines have increasing levels of resistance that you can build toward.

3. Do you have the approval of your spouse and peers? Family and friendship support systems can be a very important part of keeping your exercise program alive. A spouse's disapproval or resentment over the time you spend exercising can be very damaging to your program. Stop it before it happens, if you can. Explain to your spouse just how crucial exercise is to you (this should not be difficult with the information you now have from this book), and try to get his or her approval before you even begin. Of course, exercising together with your spouse is the best solution of all.

The most important thing to remember as you plan your approach to exercise is that the person you are trying to please in all of this is you. Don't put yourself in a position in which you'll feel uncomfortable. For example, don't begin with an advanced aerobics class if you're going to feel embarrassed about not keeping up. And again, don't be afraid to ask a professional for help. Aerobic exercise is very, very important. Your personal exercise plan must allow for thirty-minute sessions of aerobic exercise four times a week. You'll be doing this for one month before you even think about your eating problems. (It's possible that you may even begin to lose some weight during this first month. Very recent research has shown that it may be possible to lose weight through physical exercise, even without changing eating habits.)

STEP FOUR: EATING

Now, for eating. This is the last big step in the process, which you should begin after one month of an aerobic exercise program. To retrain your mind to respond to your body's physiological needs, follow these two retraining plans:

Plan 1. *Retrain yourself to respond to hunger.* Think about your hunger on a scale of one to ten. One is full, and ten is ravenous. For at least one week, do not eat unless your hunger number is greater than five. If it's less than five, then wait until it goes up before you eat. This is the only eating change you should make during the first week.

Plan 2. *Retrain yourself to respond to fullness.* In the second week, whenever you eat, stop before you're full. Wait fifteen minutes, and then if you're still hungry, eat some more. Often you'll find that after fifteen minutes you'll no longer be hungry. Spend your second week retraining yourself to eat this way. Do not worry about calories.

LOSING WEIGHT

For restrained and unrestrained eaters alike, it's now time to think about losing weight.

The first question to ask yourself is, how much? What should your goal be? You know after reading this book that the answer isn't simple. And to figure it out, you'll have to ask yourself some more questions.

1. Setpoint. What is your setpoint? While science tells us that the best weight goal is your setpoint, unfortunately we do not yet have the guidelines to tell us exactly what the setpoint number is for each of us. But you still may be able to approximate your setpoint. Was there ever a period of time in your life when you were not consciously trying to control your weight, and also not compulsively eating or gaining weight? If you can remember what your weight was during this period, you have a baseline setpoint number. Now, add five to ten pounds for each decade since then, and another five to ten pounds for each pregnancy since then. And you should have an *approximation* of your setpoint.

2. Average weight. Some people won't be able to figure out their approximate setpoint. But there are other scales that can help you determine what your new weight goal should be. The ideal weight tables can help you compare your weight to the average. Use the following table to see what your ideal body weight range is, keeping in mind the way these charts are developed (see pp. 57–60.)

You'll be surprised to find that the weight range table indicates a higher weight range than the media usually suggests. Average weights are not thin—they're average.

3. No goals. There's still another possibility to consider in figuring out your goal weight, and that's setting no goal at all! Seriously, you can guarantee success in your weight control program, if you don't have any goal holding you back. Just exercise regularly and eat sensibly, and see where you get. It's a good possibility, and it can give you immediate peace of mind. So keep it open as an option.

WHAT TO EAT

The important goal here is not to be obsessed with food or calories. Calories are obviously important, but don't cut certain foods out of your life completely. Be sensible about portions (too big and too small). Your body will tell you what it wants if you let it. There are no particular rules, just common sense. You probably already know how much food to eat to maintain your weight. Add exercise to that, and you'll lose! (See chart at the end of this chapter for some guidelines.)

As for time frames, the choice is yours. To lose weight, you only need to create an energy deficit. (If you were to create a 350,000-calorie deficit in a year, you'd lose 100 pounds.) An easy and realistic way to think about eating is by the week. On

1980 METROPOLITAN HEIGHT & WEIGHT TABLES

Weight at ages 25–29 based on lowest mortality. Weight in pounds according to frame (in indoor clothing weighing 5 pounds for men and 3 lbs. for women; shoes with 1" heels for men and women).

Courtesy of Metropolitan Life Insurance Company.

WOMEN

Feet	Height Inches	Small Frame	Medium Frame	Large Frame
4	10	102–111	109–121	118–131
4	11	103–113	111–123	120–134
5	0	104–115	113–126	122–137
5	1	106–118	115–129	125–140
5	2	108–121	118–132	128–143
5	3	111–124	121–135	131–147
5	4	114–127	124–138	134–151
5	5	117–130	127–141	137–155
5	6	120–133	130–144	140–159
5	7	123–136	133–147	143–163
5	8	126–139	136–150	146–167
5	9	129–142	139–153	149–170
5	10	132–145	142–156	152–173
5	11	135–148	145–159	155–176
6	0	138–151	148–162	158–179

MEN

Feet	Height Inches	Small Frame	Medium Frame	Large Frame
5	2	128–134	131–141	138–150
5	3	130–136	133–143	140–153
5	4	132–138	135–145	142–156
5	5	134–140	137–148	144–160
5	6	135–142	139–151	146–164
5	7	138–145	142–154	149–168
5	8	140–148	145–157	152–172
5	9	142–151	148–160	155–176
5	10	144–154	151–163	158–180
5	11	146–157	154–166	161–184
6	0	149–160	157–170	164–188
6	1	152–164	160–174	168–192
6	2	155–168	164–178	172–197
6	3	158–172	167–182	176–202
6	4	162–176	171–187	181–207

busy or less hungry days, you can build up a deficit (particularly if you limit late-night eating). On other days, you'll probably be eating more, but you still will have created a deficit for the week. This is a realistic plan. And while it may not always involve three well-balanced meals a day, it does account for the usual eating patterns of most people—on some days we simply eat more than we do on others.

If you keep up the exercise, your weight loss program will work. Don't let the scale be your guide. Rely on your own common sense, experience, and what you've learned in this book.

It will take time, but what's the rush? You have your whole life to be your normal, healthy weight, and to enjoy it!

NEW AMERICAN EATING GUIDE

Adapted from *New American Eating Guide* which is available from the Center for Science in the Public Interest, 1501 16th Street, N.W., Washington, D.C., 20036, for $3.95/$7.95 laminated, copyright 1983.

	ANYTIME	IN MODERA-TION	NOW AND THEN
Group 1 **Beans, Grains, and Nuts** *four or more servings a day*	bread and rolls (whole grain) bulgur dried beans and (legumes) peas lentils oatmeal pasta, whole wheat rice, brown rye bread sprouts whole grain hot and cold cereal whole wheat matzoh	cornbread 8 flour tortilla 8 hominy grits 8 macaroni and matzoh 8 cheese 1,(6),8 nuts 3 pasta, except whole wheat 8 peanut butter 3 pizza 6,8 refined, unsweetened cereals 8 refried beans, commercial 1, homemade in oil 2 seeds 3 soybeans 2 tofu 2 waffles or pancakes, syrup 5,(6),8 white bread and rolls 8 white rice 8	croissant 4,8 doughnut (yeast leavened) 3 or 4,5,8 presweetened breakfast cereals 5,8 sticky buns 1 or 2,5,8 stuffing, made with butter 4,(6),8

	ANYTIME	IN MODERATION	NOW AND THEN
Group 2 **Fruits and Vegetables** *four or more servings a day*	All fruits and vegetables except those listed at right applesauce (unsweetened) unsweetened fruit juices unsalted vegetable juices potatoes, white or sweet	avocado 3 cole slaw 3 cranberry sauce (canned) 5 dried fruit french fries, homemade in vegetable oil 2, commercial 1 fried eggplant (veg. oil) 2 fruits canned in syrup 5 gazpacho 2,(6) glazed carrots 5,(6) guacamole 3 potatoes au gratin 1,(6) salted vegetable juices 6 sweetened fruit juices 5 vegetables canned with salt 6	coconut 4 pickles 6
Group 3 **Milk Products** *two servings a day*	buttermilk made from skim milk lassi (low-fat yogurt and fruit juice drink) low-fat cottage cheese low-fat milk, 1% milkfat low-fat yogurt nonfat dry milk skim milk skim milk cheeses (6) skim milk and banana shake	cocoa made with skim milk 5 cottage cheese, regular, 4% milkfat 1 frozen low-fat yogurt 5 ice milk 5 low-fat milk, 2% milkfat 1 low-fat yogurt, sweetened 5 mozzarella cheese, part-skim type only 1,(6)	cheesecake 4,5 cheese fondue 4,(6) cheese soufflé 4,(6),7 eggnog 1,5,7 hard cheeses: blue, brick, Camembert, cheddar, Muenster, Swiss 4,(6) ice cream 4,5 processed cheeses 4,6 whole milk 4 whole milk yogurt 4

	ANYTIME	IN MODERA-TION	NOW AND THEN
Group 4 **Poultry, Fish, Meat, and Eggs** *two servings a day* Vegetarians: nutrients in these foods can be obtained by eating more foods in groups 1, 2, and 3	FISH cod flounder gefilte fish (6) haddock halibut perch pollock rockfish shellfish, except shrimp sole tuna, water packed (6) EGG PRODUCTS egg whites *only* POULTRY chicken or turkey, boiled, baked, or roasted (no skin)	FISH (drained well if canned) fried fish 1 or 2 herring 3,6 mackerel, canned 2,(6) salmon, pink, canned 2,(6) sardines 2,(6) shrimp 7 tuna, oil-packed 2,(6) POULTRY chicken liver, baked or broiled, 7 (just one!) fried chicken, homemade in vegetable oil 3 chicken or turkey, boiled, baked, or roasted (with skin) 2 RED MEATS (trimmed of all outside fat!) flank steak 1 leg or loin of lamb 1 pork shoulder or loin, lean 1 round steak or ground round 1 rump roast 1 sirloin steak, lean 1 veal 1	POULTRY fried chicken, commercially prepared 4 EGG cheese omelet, 4,7 egg yolk or whole egg (about 3 per week) 3,7 RED MEATS bacon 4,(6) beef liver, fried, 1,7 bologna, 4,6 corned beef 4,6 ground beef, 4 ham, trimmed well, 1,6 hot dogs, 4,6 liverwurst 4,6 pig's feet 4 salami 4,6 sausage 4,6 spare ribs 4 untrimmed red meats 4

KEY: 1–moderate fat, saturated; 2–moderate fat, unsaturated; 3–high fat, unsaturated; 4–high fat, saturated; 5–high in added sugar; 6–high in salt or sodium; (6)–may be high in salt or sodium; 7–high in cholesterol; 8–refined grains

Sources

Bennett, W., and Gurin J.: *The Dieter's Dilemma,* Basic Books, New York, 1982.

Brody, J.: *Jane Brody's Nutrition Book,* New York, Bantam Books, 1987.

Strunkurd, A.J.: *Obesity,* Philadelphia, W.B. Saunders Co., 1980.

Wurtman, R.J., and Wurtman, J.J.: *Human Obesity,* Annals of the New York Academy of Sciences, Vol. 499, New York Academy of Sciences, 1987.

Storlie, J., and Jordan, H.A.: *Behavioral Management of Obesity,* New York, Spectrum Publications, 1984.

_____: *Evaluation and Treatment of Obesity,* New York, Spectrum Publications, 1984.

_____: *Nutrition and Exercise in Obesity Management,* New York, Spectrum Publications, 1984.

Index